ON PSYCHOANALYSIS AND VIOLENCE

Psychoanalysis has not examined violence as such since it is a sociological and criminological concept; psychoanalysis is concerned with speech. *On Psychoanalysis and Violence* brings together noted Lacanian psychoanalysts and scholars to fill an important gap in psychoanalytic scholarship that addresses what the contributors term the "angwash" of our current time.

Today, violence is everywhere. We are inundated with it, exhausted by it, bombarded by images and reports of it on a daily, even hourly basis. This book examines how psychoanalysis can account for the many manifestations of violence in contemporary society. Drawing on a broadly Lacanian perspective, the authors explore violence in war, terrorism, how the media portrays violence, violent video games, questions of identity, difference and the "other"; violence narratives and violence and DSM, and explain how to account for the way violence arises and the effect it has on us on both an individual and social level. These are just some of the daily social realities of the present, whose aggression is felt by everyone, which horrifies us and which we often feel powerless to change. The contributors have therefore coined a term for this cultural malaise: "angwash", arguing that we are awash in *angoisse*, or anxiety, in a constant panic regarding the impossible and contradictory demands of a "civilization" in crisis.

On Psychoanalysis and Violence will be of great interest to Lacanian psychoanalysts and psychoanalytic psychotherapists.

Vanessa Sinclair, Psy.D. is a psychoanalyst based in New York City, USA, and Stockholm, Sweden, author of *Switching Mirrors* (Trapart, 2016) and the upcoming *Scansion in Psychoanalysis and Art: The Cut in Creation* (Routledge, 2019) and editor of *Rendering Unconscious* (Trapart, 2018).

Manya Steinkoler, Ph.D. is an English Professor at Borough of Manhattan College CUNY and a psychoanalyst in New York City, USA. She is co-editor with Patricia Gherovici of *Lacan on Madness: Madness, Yes You Can't* (Routledge, 2015), *Lacan, Psychoanalysis and Comedy* (Cambridge University Press, 2016) and forthcoming *Psychoanalysis and Sexuality: From Feminism to Trans* (Cambridge University Press, 2019).

ON PSYCHOANALYSIS AND VIOLENCE

Contemporary Lacanian Perspectives

Edited by
Vanessa Sinclair and Manya Steinkoler

Routledge
Taylor & Francis Group
LONDON AND NEW YORK

First published 2019
by Routledge
2 Park Square, Milton Park, Abingdon, Oxon OX14 4RN

and by Routledge
711 Third Avenue, New York, NY 10017

Routledge is an imprint of the Taylor & Francis Group, an informa business

British Library Cataloguing-in-Publication Data
A catalogue record for this book is available from the British Library

Library of Congress Cataloging-in-Publication Data
Names: Sinclair, Vanessa, editor. | Steinkoler, Manya, editor.
Title: On psychoanalysis and violence : contemporary Lacanian perspectives / edited by Vanessa Sinclair and Manya Steinkoler.
Description: Abingdon, Oxon ; New York, NY : Routledge, 2019. | Includes bibliographical references and index.
Identifiers: LCCN 2018030350 (print) | LCCN 2018033049 (ebook) | ISBN 9780429437342 (Master) | ISBN 9780429793769 (Web PDF) | ISBN 9780429793752 (ePub) | ISBN 9780429793745 (Mobipocket/Kindle) | ISBN 9781138346307 (hardback : alk. paper) | ISBN 9781138346338 (pbk. : alk. paper)
Subjects: LCSH: Violence—Psychological aspects. | Agressiveness. | Psychoanalysis. | Lacan, Jacques, 1901-1981.
Classification: LCC BF575.A3 (ebook) | LCC BF575.A3 O52 2019 (print) | DDC 155.2/32—dc23
LC record available at https://lccn.loc.gov/2018030350

ISBN: 978-1-138-34630-7 (hbk)
ISBN: 978-1-138-34633-8 (pbk)
ISBN: 978-0-429-43734-2 (ebk)

Typeset in Bembo and Stone Sans
by Florence Production Ltd, Stoodleigh, Devon, UK

Dedicated to Franz Kaltenbeck (1944–2018)

CONTENTS

NOTES ON CONTRIBUTORS

Judith Butler is Maxine Elliot Professor in the Department of Comparative Literature and the Program of Critical Theory at the University of California, Berkeley. She is the author of *Subjects of Desire: Hegelian Reflections in Twentieth-Century France* (1987), *Gender Trouble: Feminism and the Subversion of Identity* (1990), *Bodies That Matter: On the Discursive Limits of "Sex"* (1993), *The Psychic Life of Power: Theories of Subjection* (1997), *Excitable Speech* (1997), *Antigone's Claim: Kinship Between Life and Death* (2000), *Precarious Life: Powers of Violence and Mourning* (2004), *Undoing Gender* (2004), *Who Sings the Nation-State?: Language, Politics, Belonging* (with Gayatri Spivak in 2008), *Frames of War: When Is Life Grievable?* (2009) and *Is Critique Secular?* (co-written with Talal Asad, Wendy Brown and Saba Mahmood, 2009) and *Sois Mon Corps* (2011), co-authored with Catherine Malabou. Her most recent books include: *Parting Ways: Jewishness and the Critique of Zionism* (2012), *Dispossessions: The Performative in the Political* (co-authored with Athena Athanasiou, 2013), *Senses of the Subject* (2015) and *Notes Toward a Performative Theory of Assembly* (2015).

Guy Dana is a psychiatrist, psychoanalyst and current President of the Cercle Freudien in Paris. He was clinical director of a sector in France that included the Hospital of Barthelemy Durand, an outpatient clinic, crisis center, and therapeutic house, and ran a private psychoanalytic practice for over 40 years. He has lectured on the institutional treatment of psychosis around the world. Dana did his clinical internships with Jacques Lacan. He is the author of *Quel Politique Pour La Folie?: Le suspense de Freud* (2011), as well as hundreds of articles on psychoanalysis, both theoretical and clinical.

Todd Dean is a psychiatrist and training and supervising psychoanalyst in St. Louis, Missouri. He is a senior editor of *Division/Review* and an adjunct instructor of psychiatry at Washington University School of Medicine.

Martine Fourré is a psychoanalyst with Espace Analytique and Forums du Champ Lacanien in Paris. Today, in Dakar, she directs the center for children and adolescents as well as the center for adults that she helped found. Her books include *Les lieux d'accueil, espace social et éthique psychanalytique* (1992), *De l'érotisme comme éthique, Question sur l'amour contemporain en Occident* (1999), *L'effet Dolto. Critique raisonnée des travaux de Françoise Dolto* (2001), *L'acte du praticien et les politiques sociales* (2001), *Le deuil de l'Autre. A l'intention des psychanalystes, des travailleurs sociaux et des représentants politiques* (2002), *La folie de vivre. Quelle présence offrir au mal de vivre?* (2013), *Incasables: Parents et praticiens racontent et analysent leurs vies avec leurs enfants dit "incasables"* (2016).

Patricia Gherovici, Ph.D. is a psychoanalyst and analytic supervisor. She is co-founder and director of the Philadelphia Lacan Group and Associate Faculty, Psychoanalytic Studies Minor, University of Pennsylvania (PSYS), Honorary Member at IPTAR the Institute for Psychoanalytic Training and Research in New York City, Member at Apres-Coup Psychoanalytic Association New York and Founding Member of Das Unbehagen. Her books include *The Puerto Rican Syndrome* (Other Press, 2003), winner of the Gradiva Award and the Boyer Prize, and *Please Select Your Gender: From the Invention of Hysteria to the Democratizing of Transgenderism* (Routledge, 2010). She has published two edited collections (both with Manya Steinkoler): *Lacan On Madness: Madness, Yes You Can't* (Routledge, 2015) and *Lacan, Psychoanalysis and Comedy* (Cambridge University Press, 2016). Her new book *Transgender Psychoanalysis: A Lacanian Perspective on Sexual Difference* was published by Routledge in June 2017.

Franz Kaltenbeck (1944–2018) was a psychoanalyst active in Paris and Lille, who led the Psychoanalysis and Criminology group at the University Hospital in Lille. Dr. Kaltenbeck worked as a psychoanalyst in Séquedin, a high-security prison in the North of France. He was senior editor of the journal *Savoirs et clinique. Revue de psychanalyse*, and has published many essays in international psychoanalytic journals. His books include *Lesen mit Lacan* (*Reading with Lacan. Essays on Psychoanalysis*, Berlin, 2013) and *Reinhard Priessnitz: Der stille Rebell* (Graz and Vienna, 2006), a monograph on a Viennese poet. He co-edited *Sigmund Freud: Immer noch Unbehagen in der Kultur?* (Berlin, Zürich, 2009) and *Au-delà du deuil: Michael Turnheim* (Diaphanes, 2013). Some of his articles in English include: "The Seed of Emptiness. Melancholy of The Pale King", in *David Foster Wallace: Presences of the Other*, edited by Beatrice Pire and Pierre-Louis Patoine (Sussex Academic Press, 2017), "An Artist's Theory of Money", *Cardozo Law Review* no. 6, New York (2012) and "The Double Loss. Humour of Melancholy in David Foster Wallace's Writings" (2014).

Patrick Landman is a psychiatrist, child psychiatrist, psychoanalyst, lawyer, and senior analyst member and past president of Espace Analytique. He is President of the Initiative for a Clinic of the Subject: STOP DSM and an Associate Researcher at the University of Paris VII. He is the author of *Tristesse Business: le scandale du dsm 5* (Max Milo, 2013), *Le Refoulement Comment Pourquoi?* (Érès, 2014) and *Tous Hyperactifs?* (Albin Michel, 2016).

Vincent Le Corre is a psychologist, psychoanalyst and professor of psychoanalysis at Paris VII, Member of ALEPH, association for psychoanalysis. Le Corre has published extensively on video games and adolescence in *L'adolescent, entre marges, art et culture: une clinique des médiations en groupe* (Érès, 2013) and has many articles on clinical subjects in *Enfance et Psy, Savoir et Clinique*, CANAL psy and many other clinical and theoretical journals in France.

Juliet Flower MacCannell is Professor Emerita of English and Comparative Literature at the University of California, and since 2000 has been co-chair of the California Psychoanalytic Circle and co-editor of its publication *(a): The Journal of Culture and the Unconscious*. She formerly co-edited *The American Journal of Semiotics* with Dean MacCannell. She is the author of over 90 articles and books, among which are *Figuring Lacan: Criticism and the Cultural Unconscious* (1986/2014), *The Regime of the Brother: After the Patriarchy* (1991) and *The Hysteric's Guide to the Future Female Subject* (2000).

Todd McGowan teaches theory and film at the University of Vermont. He is the author of *Only a Joke Can Save Us: A Theory of Comedy* (2017), *Capitalism and Desire: The Psychic Cost of Free Markets* (2016), *Contemporary Film Directors: Spike Lee* (2014), *The Fictional Christopher Nolan* (2013), *Enjoying What We Don't Have: The Political Project of Psychoanalysis* (2013), *The Real Gaze: Film Theory After Lacan* (2007) and *The Impossible David Lynch* (2007).

Geneviève Morel is a psychoanalyst in Paris and Lille. She's a member of CRIMIC (Paris-Sorbonne) and CFAR (London), President of Savoirs et clinique and Collège de Psychanalystes- A.l.e.p.h. She directs a clinical seminar in l'UHSA (CHU-Lille). Her books include *Ambiguïtés sexuelles. Sexuation et psychose* (2000), published in English as *Sexual Ambiguities* (2011), *Clinique du suicide* (Érès, 2002/2010), *L'œuvre de Freud. L'invention de la psychanalyse*, (2006), *La loi de la mère. Essai sur le sinthome sexuel* (2008), published in German as *Das gesetz der Mutter* (2017) and forthcoming in English in 2017.

Jean-Jacques Moscovitz has been a practicing psychiatrist and psychoanalyst in Paris for 60 years. He is the author of *Une psychanalyse pourquoi faire?* Grancher (ed.), 1988 (new edition, September, 2006), *D'où viennent les parents? Psychanalyse depuis la Shoah?* edition L'Harmattan collection Penta, September, 2007, *Hypothèse Amour (entre intime et politique)* Calman-Lévy (ed.), 2001; *Lettre d'un psychanalyste à Steven Spielberg ou comment dé-pervertir le futur?, Shoah, le film, des psychanalystes écrivent*, Grancher (ed.), 1991 (out of print); *Rêver de réparer l'Histoire, psychanalyse cinéma politiqe*, Érès (ed.), 2015. He is a member of Espace Analytique and founding member of Psychanalyse Actuelle (1987) and directs *Le Regard qui bat*, a well-known group dedicated to cinema and psychoanalysis.

Carol Owens is a psychoanalyst and clinical supervisor in private practice in North Dublin. She has lectured on psychoanalysis at Trinity College Dublin, Dublin City University and Independent Colleges Dublin. A registered practitioner member of the Association for Psychoanalysis and Psychotherapy in Ireland, she is also the founder of the Dublin Lacan Study Group. Her work has been published in a number of journals and books.

Gérard Pommier is a psychiatrist, psychoanalyst and Director of Research at the University of Paris 7. He is Honorary Professor at the University of Rosario (Argentina). He is the director of the journal *La Clinique Lacanienne*, one of the founding members of Fondation européenne pour la psychanalyse and member of Espace Analytique. His list of books and articles is far too long to put in a paragraph. His latest works include: *Féminin, révolution sans fin* (Pauvert, 2016), *Que veut dire "faire" l'amour?* (Flammarion, 2011) and *Le nom propre* (P.U.F., 2013).

Vanessa Sinclair, Psy.D. is a psychoanalyst based in New York City and Stockholm, author of *Switching Mirrors* (Trapart, 2016) and co-editor of *The Fenris Wolf*, vol. 9 (Trapart, 2017) with Carl Abrahamsson. She recently edited a collection of psychoanalytic writing and poetry entitled *Rendering Unconscious* (Trapart, 2018) and hosts a podcast of the same name addressing the state of psychoanalysis and mental health care today, current events, culture and the arts. Her upcoming book *Scansion in Psychoanalysis and Art: The Cut in Creation* (Routledge, 2019) is part of the Art, Creativity and Psychoanalysis series edited by George Hagman. Dr. Sinclair is a founding member of Das Unbehagen: A Free Association for Psychoanalysis. She organizes events and conferences internationally, including "On Violence and Psychoanalysis: Civilization and its Bliss-contents" with Manya Steinkoler (New York City, 2015) from which this book stems.

Manya Steinkoler, Ph.D. is a practicing psychoanalyst in New York City and teaches English at Borough of Manhattan College, CUNY. She has co-edited, along with Patricia Gherovici, *Lacan on Madness: Madness, Yes You Can't* (Routledge, 2015), *Lacan, Psychoanalysis and Comedy* (Cambridge University Press, 2016) and the forthcoming *Psychoanalysis, Gender and Sexuality* (Cambridge University Press, 2019), and is an editor of *Division/Review* (New York) and *La Clinique Lacanienne* (Paris). She has completed a manuscript, *The Uncoming Community: Trauma and the Cinema of War*, with Professor Jessica Datema and has authored many articles both in English and French. She is the co-organizer along with Dr. Michael Garfinkle of *Psychoanalysis on Ice* (Reykjavik, 2014 and 2018).

Stephanie Swales, Ph.D. is an Assistant Professor of Psychology at the University of Dallas, a licensed clinical psychologist and candidate psychoanalyst in private practice in Dallas, TX. She is the founder of the Dallas/Fort-Worth area Lacan study group and the President-Elect for the Dallas Society for Psychoanalytic Psychology. Her first book, *Perversion: A Lacanian Psychoanalytic Approach to the Subject*, was published by Routledge in 2012. She has published numerous articles and chapters from a Lacanian perspective. Along with Carol Owens, she is co-authoring a book on ambivalence, which is forthcoming in early 2019.

Alireza Taheri teaches Lacanian theory as part of the Toronto Psychoanalytic Society's extension program. He is a permanent faculty member of HamAva Psychoanalytic Institute in Tehran (Iran), where he teaches psychoanalytic theory and practice, and is the book review editor of *Psychoanalytic Discourse* (an independent international journal for the clinical, theoretical and cultural discussion of psychoanalysis). He has published numerous articles in peer-reviewed journals and is currently working on a book project entitled *Specter of Madness: Reflections on the Paradoxes of Subjectivity and the Diremptions of Modernity*.

FOREWORD

Is the American youth rebelling against America?

Gérard Pommier

Just after the Stoneman Douglas High School shooting, I read the declaration of 18-year-old Emma Gonzales: "We are going to change the law." I saw the picture of David Hogg, also age 17, standing on the roof of a car, his face transfigured by his words. Perhaps the Second Amendment which gives citizens the right to bear arms to defend the security of a free state and protect themselves has nothing to do with what that "right" has become. In ancient Athens, citizens slept next to their spears; in English common law, the 1689 Bill of Rights enshrined the people's right to bear arms (in order to protect the king against a possible uprising); in Switzerland, every citizen has a war rifle under his bed, and during the French Revolution, Robespierre demanded that the right to insurrection should be included in the Constitution. However, since the roar of artillery in the 1848 and 1870 revolutions, French lawmakers have done their best to keep the people unarmed.

The history of the United States includes large strikes and violent uprisings, such as the protests and rebellions of the Civil Rights Movement and the Stonewall Riots. In 1969, Black Panthers were assassinated, having never fired a shot themselves. These 1960s revolutionaries never made use of their constitutional right to take up arms against injustice. Watching today's youth revolt, we again hear David and Emma say that they will not take up arms in order to enact change in gun control legislation.

In the course of history, the spirit of the Second Amendment has been emptied of its originary republican ferment to become justified based on the principle of "self-defense." Over the years, the Second Amendment has led to more and more spectacular crimes. America has 4.4 percent of the world's population, but nearly half of the world's civilian-owned guns. There have been 1,600 mass shootings since Sandy Hook. Since the beginning of 2018, there have already been 20 school shootings. As this book goes to press, and the editors send me this document for copy-editing, I always have to add to that number. By the time it is published, these figures will already be surpassed. According to the journal *Pediatrics*, a bullet wound is the third leading cause of death in children – every week, 25 minors die in this way.

America has its own unique form of gun madness. According to a congressional report, the number of weapons owned in the United States stands at 270–310 million where the population in 2016 was 323 million – that means a gun for every American. And hasn't anyone who owns a weapon at least thought of killing, imagined something in his head and mentally slain his enemies? Who are the enemies of the people who buy guns? Montesquieu claims that beyond the established laws of the land, we should be attentive to the "Spirit of the Laws." With that in mind, we might consider who these weapons are aimed at in the first place.

American history is symbolized by a commemoration that over time became a national holiday: Thanksgiving. When the Mayflower pilgrims landed in New Plymouth Bay in 1620, they were dying of hunger and cold. They were saved by the Wampanoag tribe, who taught them to fish and hunt, grow corn and raise turkeys, which became a staple of even the European Christmas meal. And we all know how the story continues: the Native Americans were hunted and exterminated over the next 300 years. The colonists were seized by a kind of extermination delirium, killing not just the indigenous peoples, but also buffaloes, birds and eagles, today's symbol of the United States. Do these historical facts reveal something of the "spirit" of American law? A hidden spirit, because even today the effects of this genocide have not been sufficiently recognized. There are two Thanksgivings in today's United States: the happy family holiday, which brings 3 million people to Manhattan for the Macy's parade, and the day of mourning for Native peoples.

Is murder fundamental to the "spirit" of the Law? Plymouth's Pilgrim Fathers were the carriers of an extremist religion, fundamentally similar to those that still ignite wars today. These Puritans were more Protestant than the Protestants and were fleeing England to found the "City of God" – one that would conform to the Gospel's Parable of the Sower, turned by Martin Luther into dogma. On one side we have God's Chosen, on the other the Forsaken, whom the Chosen must exterminate in order to continuously expand the "City of God." The very term "Puritan" carries within itself – no doubt unwittingly – the phantom of racial purity.

It is not enough to recognize that the National Rifle Association is a powerful lobby, one that bankrolls the American political machinery for its own benefit (as was the case with the Trump campaign, which received over $30 million from the NRA). Thanks to its influence, 65,000 gun stores (more than the number of Starbucks and McDonald's combined) can offer their arsenal for purchase. Does the NRA with its 5 million gun-slinging members not embody the spirit of the founding Puritans and their murderous delirium?

Some have called for a ban on selling weapons to the "mentally ill." However, these "mentally ill" are not as crazy as all that! They may be the most sensitive to the spirit of their nation and carry out its actions unbeknown to them; they purify the "land of the free and the home of the brave." Others have argued for the ban on automatic weapons and bump stocks. Yet these measures are no match against the onslaught of mass shootings. The same spirit will continue to blow. Only a New Spirit can rise up against the Old. Why do these mass shootings predominantly occur in schools and universities? No doubt because these are the sites of transmission, where a new rebellion against the Old Spirit of the laws might be born. A nation is great only when it knows how to sail against the wind. Isn't this the promise of Emma and David, the American youth who March for Our Lives in Washington?

On the international stage America symbolizes freedom, and Americans as individuals seem to feel a personal responsibility to take a stand for this cause. I myself am French, and share a revolutionary and republican history with my American brothers. I own a gun and a rifle, as the memory of Nazism is still fresh for a man of my generation. I remember my grandparents, Milka and Haim, murdered in Auschwitz. But today, the weapon we must arm ourselves with, as the American youth reminds us, is the New Spirit itself.

On Psychoanalysis and Violence: Contemporary Lacanian Perspectives, I hope will be a part of awakening this New Spirit.

Gérard Pommier, Paris, France 2018

INTRODUCTION

Vanessa Sinclair and Manya Steinkoler

Today, violence is everywhere. We are inundated with it, exhausted by it, *bomb*arded by images and reports of it on a daily, even hourly basis, in real time with minute-to-minute updates via "breaking news" alerts on our iPhones, constant notifications and emails. From terrorism to the "war on terrorism," from the exponential increase in mortality due to opioid overdose to "the war on drugs," from mass shootings to the helplessness felt by the impossibility of enacting protective gun legislation, from school shootings by disgruntled, neglected teens to the failure of the mental health-care system to address the often glaring warning signs, from constant coverage of the tweeter-in-chief, who regularly overturns every principle of democratic and humane tenets of government only to replace them with a tyrannical whirlwind of inappropriate, impulsive, narcissistic and highly aggressive rants to hostile contention regarding the reporting of the very facts of the news – is it fake? Is that what really happened? – the crisis in authority is just another way that we can't get rid of it, make it go away, contain it or limit our access to it. While the debate on the benefits and detriments of technology rages, our ability to concentrate and read anything longer than a headline is increasingly rare, as even professional researchers become reduced to Olympic-level scrollers, skiing on the surface of information. The reduction of education to exam preparation, the addiction of children and teenagers to violent video games and social media, the diminishment of human beings to mere fodder for markets, the demonization of the other and the concomitant "wall" "protecting" "us" from "them" are just some of our daily social realities whose aggression we feel, are horrified by and feel powerless to change. ADHD, autism, panic disorders, depression, anxiety, chronic pain, irritable bowel syndrome, restless legs syndrome, eczema, alcoholism, prescription drug addiction and fibromyalgia are just some of the new names of our cultural malaise.

Systemic violence and racism are pervasive, some have argued even fundamental, to our democracy and to the structure of institutions. What's been termed the new Jim Crow is effectively destroying families and communities, as our prison system overflows with generations of young black men. The police violence against these young black men seems to know no bounds. The constant assault on the Other: immigrants, women, the LGBTQ community, the disabled, and even the planet itself is part of our daily "aggression fatigue." No human relation or possibility of human bond is left unthreatened by increasing, invasive and pervasive social paranoia. Harvey Weinstein, Jerry Sandusky and Larry Nassar are names of the new Leviathan, a mythic monster that in our day and age has turned out to be all too real. All the while, underserved populations are continually pushed to the side and ignored. Quoting Harvard sociologist Robert Sampson, Ta-Nehisi Coates (2017) notes, "It's the myth of the American Dream that with initiative and industriousness, an individual can always escape impoverished circumstances. But what the data shows is that you have these multiple assaults on life chances that make transcending those circumstances difficult and at times nearly impossible." The American dream has become the American nightmare. There is no doubt that the United States seems to have experienced an uncanny volte-face; now with military parades and nighttime torch marches, we appear to be the bizarre incarnation of the very tyranny democracy has fought against from its earliest beginnings.

Jihadism and radicalization have replaced the love cults of the 1960s with machine guns and revisionist fundamentalist religion. Professor of psychiatry at the University of Virginia, Charlottesville, Vamik Volkan points out that this fundamentalism promotes a doctrine of "Total loyalty to the leader and to the divine text, 'removing' anxiety a member might have due to intrapsychic and interpersonal conflicts." The aim is to eradicate the unconscious as the topos of alterity since it threatens the fundamentalist credo. In the same vein, the "lone wolf terrorist" becomes a template for copycats who wish to replicate violent acts, testifying only to the violence that inhabits them. The alarming rise of the Alt-right and conservative populist movements have been given new impetus by the rise to power of tyrants, and the world has a new "Axis to grind" in the Erdogan–Duterte–Putin–Trump era.

The violence we endure extends to the past and the future, with catastrophic effects for future generations as the United States leaves the Paris accords while hurricanes, earthquakes, wildfires, mudslides and tsunamis eat away at the very ground we stand on. The recent tax legislation passed by Congress promises to mire our children and grandchildren in unremitting debt. Moreover, the erasure and denial of the past could not be more egregious as the demands of Indigenous peoples for respect of their tribal lands and burial grounds are ignored in favor of fracking and oil transport and production.

The erasure of time is part of the new neoliberal world of the sleepless 24/7 demand for work, which is only further exacerbated by the sense of timelessness that technology encourages. The new global culture, or mono-culture of sameness, has eviscerated the differences between bodies and information as we are increasingly induced to treat our neighbor as virtual matter. Reality has become virtual and life, a video game. We see this reach new levels in the recent phenomenon of "swatting," where gamers call police to report violence occurring at the hands of random others as a sort of prank call. The outcome of such a "game" can prove lethal, having recently resulted in the murder of a Wichita man by police answering such a "prank" call during the holiday season. Technology allows the fiction that one is not participating in a social group, interacting with others, but rather removed, autonomous and limitlessly powerful. This is seen in the phenomenon of cyber bullying and the concomitant increase in adolescent suicide. In a recent well-publicized case, Massachusetts teen Michelle Carter was convicted of involuntary manslaughter for egging on the suicide of Conrad Roy, her long-distance online boyfriend, by text message. "Just do it," she said, the Nike voice of the super-ego. The limitlessness that technology psychically permits and promotes alerts us to the appearance of the uncanny in classical Freudian terms, as something that should have been repressed but shows up in reality where it does not belong. This is illustrated as First Lady Melania Trump campaigns to tackle cyber-bullying, while her husband is a super-villain of the universe of cyber-bullying, threatening nuclear war while boast-tweeting about the size of his nuclear "button."

This book raises questions about violence and its relationship to the Other. This is why, in our estimation, violence can no longer be relegated to an extra-psychoanalytic concept. For Freud and Lacan, the concept of aggression is a properly psychoanalytic one. Violence, on the other hand, insofar as it is an act, remains outside of the realm of speech or subjectivity proper. At the same time, the more the "*disque-cours courrant*" – to quote Lacan's pun on discourse and "disque cours" or "running record/LP" – is one of violence, the more the subjective effects abound. Violence is no longer extra-linguistic as the super-egoic hegemony of cultural and ideological imperatives hold sway. Our title, *On Psychoanalysis and Violence*, brings to mind many properly psychoanalytic concepts: Oedipus, *Totem and Taboo*, killing Moses, aggression, sadism, masochism and, of course, the death drive. And yet, are any of these theoretical concepts actually violence? Psychoanalysis concerns itself fundamentally with speech and unconscious processes. Violence, on the other hand, concerns the act rather than the word, and while it may be talked about as violence, it has not traditionally been considered a psychoanalytic problem but rather a juridical or social one. At the same time, for Lacan, developing Freud's notion of primal repression, there is an originary violence of being subject to language. "The letter kills," Lacan tells us, following Hegel. The Real is simultaneously created and annulled by the encounter with language.

Lacan's development of the traumatic impact of language on the human follows from his close reading of Freud. Indeed, when asked whether psychoanalysis, a practice in and of language, might help render the world less violent, Freud responds to Einstein's optimism at the new theory of psychoanalysis with a categorical *no*, stating:

> You begin with the relation between Right and Might. There can be no doubt that that is the correct starting-point for our investigation. But may I replace the word 'might' by the balder and harsher word 'violence'? Today right and violence appear to us as antitheses. It can easily be shown, however, that the one has developed out of the other.

This intimacy between law, or right, and violence is the core of Freud's argument in *Civilization and Its Discontents.* We recall that Freud chose the etymologically unusual noun "*Unbehagen*" – not an easy one for translators – to describe what has been rendered in English and French respectively as discontents or malaise in civilization. *Unbehagen* is used in German only as a noun, while *Behagen* is both a noun and a verb. The Old Norse verbs *Haga* (to set up, arrange) and *Hagar* (it fits or to fit) belong to the verb *Hagan* (to protect, cherish) of Germanic origin, and etymologists think it was developed with the participation of the Old High German *Gihagan* (maintained, nourished). Etymologically, then, *Unbehagen* means (*un*) *not* set up, not arranged, not protected, not cherished, not nourished – all relating to a structural impossibility that Freud elaborates regarding civilized life.

We contend that *Unbehagen* is a word that is better suited to another era, and while underlining and capturing well the costs and failures of repression, it does not account for the psychic panic and existential disarray we experience today. Nowadays, the psychic shutdown is not due to repression but to overwhelming stimulation and constant social, political and personal demands that are categorically impossible to meet and come at us from all directions. This makes for a totalizing sense of panic, exhaustion and guilt. It is no longer enough to say in Althusserian terms that the subject of language is the subject of ideology. Today, the very integrity of speech as establishing bonds between people is at stake, as language is more and more harnessed to a culture of enjoyment. Existential anxiety is managed and maintained by ideological and capitalist demands for imaginary belonging. People feel guilty both for not doing enough sit-ups and for sitting too much – what has been termed, by Forbes, the *Huffington Post* and even the Mayo Clinic, "the new smoking." Subjective guilt, the loss of desire and ego ideals that previously supported cultural endeavor are harnessed by an ideology that is sustained by our mis-recognizing this guilt as a failure to conform to imaginary cultural injunctions. The constant tsunami of information and demand make for an erosion of the integrity of social-symbolic channels that previously helped access more intimate subjective truth. The blitzkrieg of fake news and the use of blatant lying about known facts only to assert power have made for what Masha Gessen has called "outrage fatigue."

We argue that we need a new word for our modern "*unbehagen.*" Lacan posited that anxiety was born of the lack of lack. Anxiety is a direct link with the Real and the failure of the symbolic order to sustain subjectivity in the face of the overwhelming object that threatens to destroy it. In Lacan's seminar X, *L'Angoisse* (Anxiety), he develops his own reading of Freud's "Inhibition, Symptom and

Anxiety" with the addition of what Lacan called his only worthwhile contribution to psychoanalysis, the object *a*. Lacan explains that anxiety never dupes and concerns the presence of something that is not dialectizable by language. Anxiety marks a limit – namely, the presence of the Real. This is rarely any longer "a subjective moment" that underlines the potential failure of fantasy to protect the subject from the Real. Rather, nowadays we are "*Angwashed*," flooded with anxiety as we are overtaken by the constant force of the Real.

The attacks of 9/11 inaugurated the 21st century with the word *terror*, ushering in a new "sense of an ending" – i.e., the twilight of nation states, of which the current ideological backlash is a symptom, as we bear witness to the eroding limits of advanced democracy buttressed by global capitalism and corporate greed. The popular and resounding backlash against our oxymoronic "culture of violence" is often experienced as yet another instance of violence as the #MeToo, Times Up, Black Lives Matter, and demand for protest activism overwhelm our daily lives. We are left with the sense that we need to be actively protesting and "doing something about it" all the time, which either feeds our narcissistic wish to "be good" or aliments our sense of overwhelming impotence. Indeed, identity politics has become a spurious retreat for the ego in the face of the daily barrage. This injunction to defend every group and decry all oppression becomes yet another onslaught. As a result, social discourse becomes reduced, flattened, lacking in nuance, eschewing all complexity into the most simplistic binary of good and bad. The triumph of "political correctness" as a new religion that guarantees "safe places" and averts us with "trigger warnings" is part of the very problem to which it tries to respond. The new identity and gender politics, the culture of medical and educational evaluation, the myriad and increasing diagnoses of mental illness have become the new "symbolic categories" of supposed "being" that risk perpetuating and exacerbating the divides that cause violence in the first place, placing the ego at the epicenter. Instead of opening dialogue, these identificatory categories establish imaginary boundaries that strangle discussion, internal reflection and stymie the ability to think.

René Girard in his famous book *Violence and the Sacred* underlines the social function of sacrifice as that which quells violence, and as such is constitutive of community, appeasing potential conflict. This notion of sacrifice makes a cut, like circumcision as a founding cutting away of *jouissance* due to which the social tie is invented and secured. This echoes Freud's myth in *Totem and Taboo* wherein the primal father is murdered and, as a result, sacrifice of enjoyment becomes the foundation of law. The 20th century saw this notion of sacrifice take off, and we learned that sacrifice marks at the same time, as Freud argued in *Civilization and Its Discontents*, the constant proximity between civilization and barbarism. For Hitler, in *Mein Kampf*, for example, people are "freed by nothing but sacrifice." Mid-century fascism finds new life in today's *Angwash* where we are never freed, and we never stop sacrificing.

How do we create the space that allows for thought that could make for a relation to the subject, ushering in the relief provided by speech? Walter Benjamin's critique of violence echoes something of the Freudian discovery. Benjamin explains how all contract "points toward violence." He continues, however, that "There is a sphere of human agreement that is nonviolent to the extent that it is wholly inaccessible to violence: the proper sphere of understanding, language." Slavoj Žižek has said that psychoanalysis today is the one practice that allows us the luxury *not* to enjoy. We contend that psychoanalytic thought and clinical practice can contribute to thinking through the challenges of our current moment, and we turn to Freud's reflections on war and the psychic origins of violence to situate our argument.

In his letters to Einstein, Freud writes:

> Such, then, was the original state of things: domination by whoever had the greater might – domination by brute violence or by violence supported by intellect. As we know, this régime was altered in the course of evolution. There was a path that led from violence to right or law. What was that path? It is my belief that there was only one: the path which led by way of the fact that the superior strength of a single individual could be rivalled by the union of several weak ones. "*L'union fait la force.*" Violence could be broken by union, and the power of those who were united now represented law in contrast to the violence of the single individual. Thus we see that right is the might of a community. It is still violence, ready to be directed against any individual who resists it; it works by the same methods and follows the same purposes. The only real difference lies in the fact that what prevails is no longer the violence of an individual but that of a community. But in order that the transition from violence to this new right or justice may be effected, one psychological condition must be fulfilled. The union of the majority must be a stable and lasting one. If it were only brought about for the purpose of combating a single dominant individual and were dissolved after his defeat, nothing would have been accomplished. The next person who thought himself superior in strength would once more seek to set up a dominion by violence and the game would be repeated ad infinitum. The community must be maintained permanently, must be organized, must draw up regulations to anticipate the risk of rebellion and must institute authorities to see that those regulations – the laws – are respected and to superintend the execution of legal acts of violence. The recognition of a community of interests such as these leads to the growth of emotional ties between the members of a united group of people – communal feelings which are the true source of its strength.

Our book aims to revitalize, renew and encourage this strength, bringing together psychoanalysts and psychoanalytic scholars to address, explore and interrogate our current cultural moment from a psychoanalytic viewpoint that is non-moral, non-putative and non-identificatory in its theorization and conceptualization. The field of psychoanalysis is just as rife as any other field with debate, theoretical disagreement and conceptual antagonism. At the same time, the possibility of thinking psychoanalytically about the problem of violence is an occasion for our diverse group of international clinicians and scholars to rally together, an example of the strength in community that Freud contends is the albeit fragile bulwark against tyranny.

We open the volume with some reflections of the French psychiatrist, psychoanalyst, analysand and student of Lacan, Jean-Jacques Moskovitz. Moskovitz writes that he is called upon to respond to the question we asked him when inviting him to contribute to our book – namely, "Why do we kill?" He argues that the *jouissance* involved in murder annihilates not only the life of the victim, but aims at annihilating the unconscious of both the murderer and the victim as the constitutive site of difference. Using Freud's theory of primal repression and the mythic murder of the father that founds the unconscious, Moskovitz is able to contrast the symbolic coordinates of human existence by opposing them to the demand for *jouissance* necessitated by ideologies of destruction. Well known for his work in Paris on cinema and psychoanalysis, Moskovitz shows how cinema can be a way of reestablishing symbolic links as well, and it is particularly well situated to constructing, *après coup*, testimony as symbolic death or inscription. Reading Lanzmann's *Shoah* and Nemes's *Son of Saul*, Moskovitz incites his readers to rally, act and bear witness to defend the integrity of the symbolic register.

The inherent contentiousness of the symbolic register is addressed as famed philosopher and gender theorist Judith Butler delineates the effects that Freud has had on philosophical and political thought. In Freud's "Thoughts for the times on war and death" (1915), written six months after the outbreak of World War I, he reflects on the bonds that hold communities together as well as the destructive powers that break them apart. By the time he develops the death drive in 1920, Freud becomes increasingly concerned with the destructive capacities of human beings. He addresses the dangers of nationalism, the phantasmatic characteristics of citizenship, the problem of authority, the origins of violence and war, and the dim prospects for peace. Butler points out that at work in Freud is an operative metaphor of the psyche as a legal system unto itself, passing judgment, asserting authority, banishing foreign elements and meting out forms of punishment. Butler's contribution underlines that the psychic sphere is already political, and that the distinctly human capacity for destructiveness follows from the ambivalent psychic constitution of the human subject. Freud is clearly looking to find a possibility in the life of the drives to counter the horrific destructiveness that he saw in World War I. Reflection on how best to avert destruction must do something other than provide an argument acceptable to rational thought; it must somehow appeal to the drive, or find a way of working with – and against – that propulsive destructiveness that can lead to war.

Literary and psychoanalytic scholar Juliet Flower MacCannell reminds us that Freud's pessimism was mitigated by his thoughts regarding the life-preserving drives. She looks at the Freud–Einstein correspondence, "Why War?," with the horrors of the recent events in Charlottesville in mind. She reflects upon the new audacity of the Alt-right and Trump's outrageous response – "very fine people on both sides." MacCannell notes that Freud sees the aim of law as binding us to the erotic and life-preserving drives, with the expressed purpose of uniting and protecting the social body. Freud demonstrates that the law developed out of violence and represents the triumph of the "might of the community" over brute force. Freud's aim, he explains to Einstein, and the aims of psychoanalysis in general, concern a transformation of the psyche, of mentality itself. MacCannell shows how this transformation is antithetical to the aims of the new administration where the triumph of the "celebration of violence" is presented as trumping the law and is instituted as a kind of imposter of the law. She shows that the Alt-right "demonstration" in Charlottesville was not a demonstration in the name of the law, but a literal *demonstration* – a parade of imaginary power, vaunting the "muscular superiority" of the Alt-right. MacCannell uses the images and chants of the Alt-right to reveal a movement based solely on the power of posturing, whose intent is to show that violence and destruction trump any gesture towards preservation and community. Like Moskovitz's contention that violence concerns the eradication of the unconscious, she underlines that this constant propping up of a violent imaginary serves to "eliminate the idea of a psyche." The Alt-right and similar reactionary right-wing movements aim at turning Freud's end of war into "endless war." MacCannell utilizes Arendt's discussion of "robotic violence" to illustrate the wish to eliminate the subject altogether, diagnosing our current moment with recourse to Arendt's famed critique of totalitarianism.

Preeminent professor of Lacanian and film theory Todd McGowan addresses the evolution of violence in our society in terms of the development of technology. Citing Foucault, Agamben and Esposito, as well as analyzing several films of Buñuel, McGowan notes the shift from punishment to discipline, and from discipline to security, as modalities of biopower. Today, overt forms of violence have been exchanged for the more subtle and insidious, as the surveillance of private behavior has trumped the dissuasive quality of the public execution. Addressing the dismissal of sexuality in Foucault's original theory, McGowan asserts that today desire and sexuality need to be reinstated more than ever. In the regime of biopower, the inherent violence and control work their way into the maintenance of life as a means and end in themselves. Subjects no longer go on living but must monitor and preserve their vitality at all costs. The survival of the biological body has become more important than the life of the subject or restraining *jouissance*. McGowan claims that in order to eroticize life and make it worth living, every regime of biopower must have recourse to death. Death comes in a wide variety of forms: horror or suspense films, health warnings about the dangers of particular foods, news coverage of natural disasters, mass shootings, and so on. The presentation of the daily bombardment of threats focuses on life itself and not on the political or social coordinates that condition or create the threat, as if these threats were akin to natural disasters rather than to political or social problems.

Mass shootings today can certainly seem like natural disasters, since they appear to be relentless and we seem to have no control over them or warning as to when they might occur. We've had 18 school shootings in the first six weeks of 2018. In recent years, there have been countless mass shootings in public places: from a nightclub in Orlando to an outdoor concert in Las Vegas; from a movie theater in Aurora, Colorado, to churches in Sutherland Springs, Texas and Charleston, South Carolina; the list goes on and on. Since Manya Steinkoler first presented her paper addressing Adam Lanza and the shooting at Sandy Hook elementary school, the frequency of school and mass shootings has snowballed, and seems an almost daily occurrence. Steinkoler examines this phenomenon through a psychoanalytic lens. Rather than participating in the popular social science notion that shooters belong to a "group" and can be identified in terms of shared criminal characteristics, she examines the case of Adam Lanza in depth to argue for more careful attention to children in distress, the signs of which are always present if we want to notice them. The Newtown shootings, where 20 children, ages 6 and 7, and 6 caretakers were killed in 2012, touched the nation and the world. Yet neither stricter gun control laws nor more rigorous protocols for the treatment of psychotic children have been put in place as a result. Steinkoler tracks Adam Lanza's story and shows how the system instituted to protect Adam, failed him. The case is important for clinicians who treat psychotic children since it shows where the clinician can go wrong while ostensibly trying to support the work. It also illuminates the problem of authority as just one of the difficulties therapists confront when working in a consumer society like the United States and dealing with psychotic children. Finally, in an apostrophe to Fritz Lang's (1931) *M*, she wonders about Adam's fascination, as well as society's, with the "child murderer" and the group tendency, so elegantly depicted by Lang, to demonize rather than understand.

A shocking number of children today are subjected from an early age to the most unspeakable violence: mistreatment, abuse, torture, involuntary and voluntary manslaughter. Franz Kaltenbeck, a French psychoanalyst who led the Psychoanalysis and Criminology group at the University Hospital in Lille and worked as a psychoanalyst in Séquedin, a high-security prison in the North of France, addresses this in his chapter on the tortured child. Assessing the National Institute of Health and Medical Research (INSERM) numbers in 2013, Anne Tuzs estimates that "two children on average . . . die every day from violence inflicted by adults, usually by their parents." They become prey to the perverted, destructive drive of adults. Some children are pampered, adored by the blind love and devotion of their parents, even idealized and cosseted, while others are abused and/or neglected. But whether adored or abused, children can rapidly lose their human status. Outlawed, they become beings whose bodies and lives are completely dependent upon the whims of their fathers, mothers or other relatives. Unfortunately, nobody will intervene in their lives and inescapable fates. Uncles, aunts, grandparents and neighbors often do not see the injuries caused by beatings: the bruises, open wounds or scars. Father, mother, brother, sister, friends . . . all too often not one of these symbolic names or social links work to protect or care for these children.

In popular culture, we often hear that children turn violent for a whole host of societal reasons, and video games are often blamed. In "Click and Destroy:

Video Games in Clinical Work," using Lacanian conceptual tools, French psychoanalyst Vincent Le Corre tries to imagine the video game as an object from a psychoanalytic point of view. He links together the concept of narcissism in terms of the mirror stage, as well the way it is revisited during puberty and adolescence together with the video game. To what extent is the violence often associated with video games a consequence of their use? Is the popular conception that compulsive gaming causes violence true? What is the cause of the violence? Is gaming a cause or a result? Developing and elaborating the concept of narcissism during adolescence allows us to view these popular assumptions more Le Corre asks what purposes video games serve. Why do individuals devote themselves to video games with such enthusiasm, or even compulsion, to the point of playing during all their waking hours? The answer to that question cannot simply consider video gaming as yet another substance on the list of the new myriad of addictions. An outgrowth of the computing world, video games are strongly linked with the symbolic realm. Therefore, Le Corre explores the various forms of pleasure and *jouissance* that a subject can procure via the cybernetic apparatus. Le Corre considers this *jouissance* with recourse to a clinical case.

Further considering the problem of violence and children, French psychoanalyst Martine Fourré theorizes violence as a "desperate call for an impossible presence," and discusses the function of the father, not simply as a metaphor that manages the mother's desire, as Lacanians are wont to repeat, but in terms of a real "authorizing" of a child that allows him to make his way in the world. Fourré's long career treating psychotic and behaviorally challenged children in the tradition of the Mannonis and Le Forts has allowed her a lifetime of experience dealing with aggression, acting out, and maladaptive behavior in infants, children and adolescents. With recourse to clinical cases and reference to several "lone wolf terrorists," Fourré underscores the foundational and salubrious function of the social link and the role of fathers in facilitating this achievement for their children. She impugns institutional violence, a false stand-in for the father, as a kind of unthinking administrative machine that "forecloses the human question" in the name of efficiency and the ideal where human beings are "reduced to objects at the expense of subjectivity." Using several popular novels and films as reference points, in addition to emphasizing the crucial function of the shared symbolic systems of storytelling and myth, Fourré underlines the need to understand and bear repetition, however chaotic, in clinical work. She reminds us that the Germanwings suicide pilot, Andreas Lubitz, sought help 41 times from clinical workers before his tragic act. The clinician has a role to support the formulations of the unconscious, as well as what has to be repeated, precisely because it cannot yet become unconscious. It is in this way that Fourré emphasizes that analysis preserves the social link; it brings the real to the possibility of language, and the torment that affects the subject "in his flesh" can be borne, and perhaps spoken.

French psychiatrist and psychoanalyst Patrick Landman, the leader of the STOP DSM movement, offers a scathing critique of the *Diagnostic and Statistical Manual of Mental Disorders* (DSM) as an ideological and institutional barrier to mental health. He shows how there is a violence in symbolic interpolation and "evaluation" that denies and can even foreclose subjective experience, impeding the very possibility of a psychoanalytic cure. Landman goes into the history of the DSM and of diagnosis of mental illness before the DSM, bringing to light the relationship between segregation and psychiatric diagnosis that has evolved over time, and insisting that the violence of psychiatric diagnosis is correlated with its segregative dimension. Landman delineates how the former model of psychiatric diagnosis with racist and colonialist accents gave way to a psychiatric diagnosis induced by pharmacology, and, as a consequence, to the hope that the naturalization of mental illness as a disease of the brain would put an end to the segregation of the mentally ill. This hope has vanished and the disappearance of psychiatry will not put an end to the peculiarity of mental illness and the segregative violence that many patients still suffer.

From the position of both American psychoanalyst and psychiatrist, Todd Dean discusses his experience working with refugees at a mental health clinic in St. Louis, and the violence inherent in the bureaucratic gymnastics required in order to treat these patients. Dean recounts that in this clinic providers are instructed to limit their work to three-month cycles of "intake forms" and mandated mental health questionnaires. The direction of treatment is completely taken out of the hands and better judgment of the clinician and placed in the bureaucratic system. As Dean states, "Algorithms have become the replacement for thinking in our world." Through clinical material, Dean addresses pervasive problems in our mental health-care system, as well as their relation to the criminal "justice" system and Immigration and Customs Enforcement. Dean demonstrates the violence of diagnosis in the search for "truth," highlighting the problems inherent in applying universals to particular situations, especially in the case of applying static measures to something as fluid as a subject's inner life. "Whatever value for bookkeeping or population statistics diagnostic inventories and manuals may have, they are alienating for the subject, every time, because they are static and therefore precluded from discourse." As Dean's clinical examples demonstrate, this is particularly clear and problematic when dealing with lives that have been affected by the trauma of war, dislocation, attempted relocation and assimilation, only to have the foundation ripped out from under them once again.

Psychiatrist, psychoanalyst and President of Cercle Freudien Guy Dana continues the discussion of clinical work with traumatized, depressive and psychotic patients on an institutional level. Dana has been concerned with the psychoanalytic treatment of serious mental illness, from his early days as an intern under Lacan's direction to becoming the director of the psychiatric Barthelemy Durand Hospital where he invented and instituted a psychoanalytic modality of working with psychotic patients. In his contribution to this volume, he critiques the word "violence" as an occasion for associative and affective logorrhea, and argues that the word itself obscures a conceptual difficulty. Violence is a word that concerns the social realm, and Dana contrasts violence with aggressivity, a properly psycho-analytic term that concerns the subject. Dana looks at violence from a clinical perspective in terms of the contemporary need for "security," not least with regard to the seriously mentally ill, and shows that "violence erupts when there is no space for associations." He sees violence as what closes down the psyche and inhibits elaboration. The work of psychoanalysis constructs an address, yet this is less frequent nowadays, and as a result we encounter more violence. Yet Dana does not stop at this initial binary; he shows that psychoanalytic practice as well as psychoanalytic institutional practice has to interrogate its own violence. Dana extends his critique to our historical moment: we live in "real time" in the media age, a time that structurally and functionally is in opposition to elaboration and to the work of the unconscious. He considers Winnicott's notion of the insufficient holding environment and uses Lacan's idea to critique Winnicott's supposed insufficiency, showing that the foundations of paranoid knowledge lurk in every person's early dependency. Reversing Winnicott's position, he shows that the first violence is of the other.

Confronting the ambivalence toward the other through the lens of television and film, Irish Lacanian psychoanalyst Carol Owens and American psychoanalyst Stephanie Swales consider the zombie. Owens and Swales claim that the inevitable tensions of ambivalence, as well as the experience of *hainamoration* itself are increasingly foreclosed under neoliberalism. This paradoxical operation accordingly produces specific effects: the return of what is foreclosed finds expression in violent zombie massacres and also operates to imbue the figure of the zombie with all our foreclosed ambivalence towards our neighbor. Žižek has commented at length on the enforcement of today's neoliberal tolerance, making use of Freud's and Lacan's insistence on the problematic nature of the basic Judeo-Christian injunction "love thy neighbor," fully bringing out the attendant obsessive fear of harassment that accompanies liberal tolerance. The evolution of the argument put forward by Owens and Swales is illuminated through cinema and in relation to the shifts in political tone from the 1960s to 1970s to today. Owens and Swales posit that pre-9/11, the foreclosure of ambivalence resulted in the return of the ambivalent figure as a "zombie" from another dimension, and that post-9/11, the neoliberal disavowal of ambivalence has produced its perverse counterpart – the "zombie" next door.

Just as the neighbor can turn into a zombie, the "girl next door" can become a jihadist or a suicide bomber. French Lacanian psychoanalyst Geneviève Morel considers why some turn towards radicalization, Islamic fundamentalism and terrorism. Morel reads the autobiographies and notes of anarchists and terrorists, wondering how a terrorist becomes a writer. In particular, she looks at the case of Susan Stern via her memoirs. She notes a tie with other terrorists in terms of the importance of ideals and of the ego ideal. Morel asks what people are doing when they seek out extremist violence. The history of the Weathermen is situated in the activism and social movements of the 1960s, where Susan Stern's story takes place. Morel notes the importance of the group and group identity for such subjects, as was the case with Stern who writes of her rebirth through the group and the loss of her ego. Stern gives herself the name "Sham," in obedience to her punishing super-ego. In her adherence to the group, she sacrifices everything in the hopes of a mythic rebirth through the ideal image of the feminist revolutionary.

The aim of the radical to annihilate conflict in search of the ideal is visited on a theoretical axis by Iranian Lacanian scholar Alireza Taheri, who considers the way that apparent contraries such as religion and atheism, masculinity and femininity, good and evil, truth and lies (to name a few) only appear opposed through an operation of misrecognition called subreption. Starting from Hegel's premise, according to which it is "an excessive tenderness for the world to keep contradiction away from it," and moving through the theories of Freud, Lacan, Kant, Žižek and Copjec, Taheri expands on the concept of subreption, positing that the failure to reckon with identities-in-difference (a failure consequent upon the operation of "subreption") relegates the subject to deeper contradictions that define central aspects of our contemporary predicament. He explains that in an ideal point we can never reach, reason (the capacity to grasp the paradox of identity-in-difference) and understanding (the faculty that misrecognizes that paradox) coincide. In other words, the misperception by which, for example, true religiosity – e.g., Hegel's notion of Christianity – and atheism are opposed, harbors a kernel of truth regarding their identity. Taheri recalls that for Lacan, "there is no truth that, in passing through awareness, does not lie." If truth and lies mask a secret identity, then the errors of understanding are perhaps our only means to access the truths of reason.

In the final chapter, Lacanian psychoanalyst Patricia Gherovici explores the possibility of psychoanalysis as resistance to violence. She examines the case of Argentina during the "Dirty War," a period of devastating state violence and human rights violations, and the concomitant rise of Lacanian psychoanalysis. Was the emergence of Lacanian psychoanalysis the effect of a political response to state violence, or did it function as a remedy that ended up being complicit with the very violence it tried to oppose? The case of Argentina offers us some insights regarding the relationship between psychoanalysis and violence. Lacan's provocative thesis that "The unconscious is structured like a language" means that the psychoanalytic subject is immersed in a universe ruled by desire and determined by a social order ushered in by language acquisition. If the formation of symptoms results from the singular structure of the subject's individual and cultural history, Lacanian psychoanalysis will be concerned with what meaning is betrayed by signs stemming from the social structure. In other words, by making symptoms readable, psychoanalysis deciphers their message at both a subjective and societal level. It brokers an integration and interrogation of the social and psychological realm. Lacanian psychoanalysis flourishes in Argentina because it integrates and addresses the multiple forms of violence present, revealing the unconscious as political by highlighting the death-drive. This chapter illuminates how violence reveals the unconscious as political, insofar as it is the discourse of the Other, and therefore can flourish in a society where repressive violence has been rife. One might conclude that psychoanalysis provides a clinico-political response to oppression and violence.

References

Alexander, M. (2010). *The New Jim Crow: Mass Incarceration in the Age of Colorblindness.* New York: The New Press.

Arendt, H. (1970). *On Violence.* New York: Harcourt.

Coates, T. (2017). *We Were Eight Years in Power: An American Tragedy.* New York: One World Publishing.

Crary, J. (2015). *24/7 Late Capitalism and the Ends of Sleep.* London: Verso.

Freud, S. (1930). Civilization and Its Discontents. *The Standard Edition of the Complete Psychological Works of Sigmund Freud (S.E.)* XXI. London: Hogarth Press. pp. 59–145.

——. (1932). *Why War? S.E.* XXII. London: Hogarth Press.

Lawrence, B. and Karim, A. (eds.). (2007). *On Violence: A Reader.* Durham, NC: Duke University Press.

Leo, G. (ed.). (2017). *Fundamentalism and Psychoanalysis.* Lecce, Italy: Frenis Zero Press.

Žižek, S. (2008). *Violence.* London: Profile Books.

1

BODIES AND THE OBJECT-DEATH

Jean-Jacques Moscovitz

I was asked to write something on the topic of – drumroll please – "Why we kill." Is this a psychoanalytic question, one that can be analyzed using our conceptual toolkits as practitioners of Freud's discovery? Or is it a political one, and should we think of it in political terms, especially following the massacre of November 13, 2016, the day of the ISIS attacks on Paris, just to mention one of many.

This is the question I was asked when approached to pen a chapter for this volume. In my book *Rêver de réparer l'histoire* (The Dream of Repairing History, 2015), I tried to link together psychoanalysis, cinema and politics by looking at a series of films and discussing several Freudian and Lacanian concepts. Surely such a link exists, because for the last 30 years I have been going on – abundantly, clumsily, insistently and, according to some, with great stubbornness – about the impact of the Shoah on our subjectivity, even before publishing, in 1991, *D'où viennent les parents, psychanalyse depuis la Shoah* (Where Parents Come From: Psychoanalysis since the Shoah).

To start off, here is Freud's conclusion to his "Thoughts for the times on war and death" (1915): "It is, to be sure, a mystery why the collective units should in fact despise, hate and detest one another – every nation against every other – and even in times of peace."

Bodies and the object-death

First, the body. In 1976, in *Joyce le symptôme*, Seminar XXIII, Lacan speaks about history, which he perceives from the perspective of an artist, himself traversed by the Symbolic of the time, and its points of fracture:

> Joyce rejects that anything can happen in what the history of historians is supposed to take for its object. He's quite right, history being nothing more

> than a flight, none of which is told but the exoduses. Through his exile, he [Joyce], sanctions the seriousness of his judgment. Deportees alone take part in history: since man's got a body, it's by the body that he can be got. The flipside of *habeas corpus*.

Habeas corpus comes from the legal Latin *habeas corpus ad subjiciendum*, which means that you have to bring your body before the judge. An institution originating in 12th-century England and codified in 1679, the Habeas Corpus Act guaranteed individual liberties of all citizens, protecting them against arbitrary arrests and detentions.

To fight against the darkness into which we are cast by torturers and barbarism, I would like to argue that with regard to the victim – the unarmed civilian targeted by genocide – every effort is made to annihilate his desire. We should understand this as a desire to kill, because the psyche, the Freudian unconscious, is the very site of murder. As psychoanalysts, we can understand this desire as the desire for the symbolic murder of the father.

Death/murder – an object (a)

Once this desire has been extinguished in the victim, they can no longer put up any resistance, much less launch a counterattack, consciously or otherwise. This is a form of silencing inherent in the desire to kill, which the criminal provokes in the victim's unconscious. Death by murder, the collective murder of one group by another, becomes an object, an object *petit a*, an object deduced between the victim and the killer. Let's take the object-gaze as an example, a very trivial one. The gaze between two fellow human beings defines the grip between two interlocutors; based on the desire to see and be seen, it becomes the cause for the desire to speak. Object a concerns a lack. However, in mass crime, the collective instead provokes an imitation of one human being by another, a reflection of the act committed by the collectively organized killer(s) against a group of victims.

By lifting the prohibition against killing, death by murder becomes available for consumption and in turn engenders the desire for more murder. The perpetrator abolishes his own internal construction of what it means to kill, rendering the act of killing a mere action without prohibition; this message is then received by the victim. The latter no longer perceives his own desire for murder and neither can he recall the very existence of the foundational prohibition against killing.

The genocidal system

The genocidal system knows this very well; this is its *raison d'être*. Mass murder is committed by one human being against another and spreads as a murderous *jouissance* that constantly reproduces itself. This annullation, this engineered removal of the knowledge of the prohibition against killing, is the production of a constructed and willful ignorance on the side of the perpetrator, which in turn provokes a silence and a silencing, a paralysis on the side of the victim. For the latter, this results in a forclusive abolition (*abolition forclusive*): the victim can no longer do anything but ignore the murderous desire present in the other, even though the latter murders with such confidence and his offence receives such widespread recognition.

Before, during and after the crime, the victim can no longer access his desire to kill, which is structurally inherent to the act of wishing to live. In a sense, the end of the fantasy of killing and being killed is equivalent to the murder of death. In this way, the genocidal killer brings his victim into his murderous world. We must keep this in mind – and teach it in the appropriate institutions to prevent the hatred against the state and its militia, which the genocidal killer is so good at fomenting. We must bring the victims out of the world of the killers, so that their death can really be their own.

This is the ethical and humanizing aim that is transmitted to us by Claude Lanzmann's film *Shoah*. Making the film was Lanzmann's way of showing how humans kill other humans. The final solution was to kill. But the word Shoah, which we use to connote the murder of the Jews, designates both the carrying out of these crimes as well as the burial of each of the Jewish victims killed in the gas chambers. This term, the title of Lanzmann's movie, attempts to return death to its place.

László Nemes's *Son of Saul* (November, 2015) is also an act of cinematic creation, a *mise-en-scène*. The unfolding drama tells the story of a member of the *Sonderkommando* in Auschwitz, some of whom were in charge of taking the men, women and children to the gas chamber where they were to be killed, and others worked in the crematorium. One child is taken from the gas chamber unconscious but still breathing and, after being examined, is then killed by a Nazi doctor. The hero of the film cannot ignore this murder and takes the child's body, literally carrying him on his shoulders, now no longer carrying out the task of murder, but taking on the symbolic burden of this son, affirming life by giving him a proper burial outside the camp, outside of the world of the killers. The Symbolic's hold over the Real of our times is embodied in this scene and in this act. We must be able to say this to our politicians whether in words or act, if we are ever to break out of this mounting violence and destruction that affects the human race and the planet we live on.

My hypothesis, which is sustained by this dimension of the Symbolic, attempts to ensure that, in the unstoppable marching of time, life triumphs over death instantiated by murder. The point is not to understand "why we kill" but to recognize the effects of these murders on the social body and its suffering in our present time.

At the moment, my hypothesis derives from Freud's key postulate of the father's murder, as described in *Moses and Monotheism* (1938). In this essay, Freud presents the crucial argument of his discipline – namely, the murder of Moses by his own people. The murdered Moses returns in the human conscience, yet his death has been repressed and remains outside consciousness. What returns is

Moses's presence as the Only God, while his murder remains unknown. Freud's point is that a repressed murder created the unconscious.

This is an example of what Freud calls "primal repression." Freud developed his hypothesis by making the signifier "Jews" the subject of the story. In his reading of the Exodus, he says that the Jews preferred to kill Moses rather than remembering that they had already killed a primal father before him. He argues that humankind has always known about this repressed foundational murder, the murder of a great man that comes prior to all others. In his essay, he calls this *an archaic heritage*. Yet the idea is already present in *Interpretation of Dreams* as early as 1900 where it is signified by the missing link in the dreamer's free associations which originate in the unconscious. Going back to the origin of speech, the narrative eventually runs into a gap, a hole, a radical lack of representation. This hole exerts an attraction; it acts as a ballast to human speech, which organizes itself around this primal lack, in other words, the Real. The origin is attached to this Real; it has to be empty. This empty place is the origin of the Symbolic voided of all Imaginary content. It functions as a border to primal repression.

Freud says very clearly that primal repression is not a clinical fact but an assumption, a logical antecedence. It is the foundation of the individual subject and of humanity, which originates from the Father's symbolic murder, the site of absence radically separate from mortal men, who are nevertheless originally connected to each other through its lack.

In terms of structure, this origin of the Symbolic translates into the "incorporation," since time immemorial, of the Father's death. It is also the recognition of the existence of death on the conscious and secular level.

This recognition constitutes the opposition between psychoanalysis and religion: all religions are founded upon such a murdered father, but only on the condition that the murder remains forgotten. Hence, the punishment by death of those who attack the religion's origin, which it believes to be its own private business, because it is directly derived from the murder of Moses, Christ, Mohammed and others. For religion, this state of ignorance must be maintained by any means.

A murder signifies an act of cutting that founds the origin of a people, which does not suppose conscious knowledge, and carries the seal of primal repression. Religion is thus founded collectively on the condition that this repression becomes the mystery or sacred enigma.

Politics and religion are connected insofar as this originary repression creates the hole in knowledge about an origin, about the foundations of human social life. The origin has to remain a void, empty of any certainty, except for what can be attributed to divine revelation. Such a postulate cannot, of course, be accepted by everyone – those who do not accept it are called infidels. Infidels are threatened by death; whether and to what degree this threat is carried out, depends on the specific religion, region and historical period.

The attacks of the Islamic State in Paris suggest that these terrorists unknowingly identify with the Real of the origin. They are not *at* the origin, the way the totalitarian regimes already familiar to us would have wished to be; instead, they *are* the origin itself. They are death in the Real, which has become the murder of both themselves and their victims. The act of killing is a deadly incest, leaving the bodies of the kamikaze intermingled with those of their victims. The ISIS (is-is, a kind of name of being, a reduced "I am that I am") takes itself for the origin of the world and immediately tries to destroy it via an apocalypse, in which the extermination of those who enjoy life is both the goal and a means to bringing an end to the human world.

This is no longer the void that all totalitarian regimes, religious or secular, want to fill with something concrete and visible, where they need to celebrate their power by excluding the bodies and words that do not fit in the world they wish to rule. For ISIS, the goal is to destroy origins, all origins. In this sense, their actions resemble a "new and improved" form of Nazism. In Germany, Death was the Master. Nazism was the previously unknown figure that destroyed everything that did not fit the shape of the origin of the humankind it invented. Everything that was not of the order of the visible, all that could have a double meaning, all equivocation, all that had to do with speaking, had to be annihilated. It was a kind of eugenics of the Symbolic itself.

For the Nazis, the Jew embodies something that cannot fit into their "models," rather, he is the source of an interpretation of their limits. Hence, the need to exterminate the Jewish people and delete the traces of this very operation, an operation that marked an imaginary border. The Nazis attempted to murder death itself and the effects of this continue to be felt by us to this day.

The appropriation of the origin

As well as being the *Fuhrerprinzip* of Nazism, this appropriation of the human origin, both individually and collectively, is the hallmark of all religions. The origin is the sphere of the gods, of one God or of many gods. In any case, religions are founded on a murder.

Today, in order to try and put an end to the acting out of the anti-state hatred and its destructive power in our world, we must be familiar with the newly recognized human rights and international institutions created during and after World War II. Today, the latter are at an unprecedented risk of becoming obsolete, given the impact on human existence, on human life and death, because the scars are so indelible, so active and so impossible to put into words.

Malraux

We must bear witness to what has happened to life, death, the law, history and the world as the integrity of the Symbolic is continually attacked. Is this really happening before us, or is it a dream that we can bear witness and that this bearing witness matters? Is this just a naive illusion of psychoanalysts, historians, citizens and artists? Our justice is called to account for itself before the tribunal of human speech. After the crimes of the Shoah and those of our time, even if it is in vain, we are confronted with a silencing and an exhaustion that burdens our minds and saps our zest for life and love.

I think that the paradigm we can identify in the Symbolic of our time is the kind of interest in otherness that we saw in the late 19th century, of otherness freed from religion and providing a place of address for liberated speech. Freud was already part of this moment writing *Interpretation of Dreams*. Malraux continued this trend, in his own way, in 1955 when he writes:

> The balance sheet of psychoanalysis shows that psychology in the past 50 years has put back the monsters and demons into man. I think that given the most terrible threat that humanity has faced, the task of the next century will be to put back the gods.

Malraux speaks at length about the developments in the Arab–Muslim world. His famous prophecy dates from 1953: "The 21st century will be religious, or it will not be at all." Just to make sure we understand this remark, Malraux is talking about the bomb. And there we have it, the theme of the question that inspired my contribution to this volume, which comes back to us today in force.

The Islamic State is here, bringing with it a cultural war against the West, annihilation and the end of the world, proclaiming the apocalypse, the extermination of the Yezidis and many other peoples, reminding us of the Nazi acts of depopulation. In this case, there is no Holocaust denial, no need for secret enjoyment, no need to lie to the victims about their fate. Quite the contrary: their mass crimes are openly exhibited, celebrated and posted all over social media. It is clear that this affirmative stance, as a counterpoint to denial, in no way prevents their threats from being carried out. The inaction of the United Nations is deafening as the question "Why we kill" always arrives much too late.

This means that alongside the movements of emancipation, whose tradition psychoanalysis reclaims, we also see, almost as a rule, the weakening of the Symbolic of our time by the destructions of humankind taking place around the world, an insistent return after we saw them in the horrors of Nazified Europe. This requires us to identify the consequences of the different discourses we engage in, listen to and that make up our everyday lives, in order to suggest actions, possible and urgent, both to our decision-makers and for ourselves.

References

Freud, S. (1900). *The Interpretation of Dreams. The Standard Edition of the Complete Psychological Works of Sigmund Freud* (*S.E.*) IV–V. London: Hogarth Press. pp. x–627.

——. (1913). *Totem and Taboo* (*S.E.*) XIII. London: Hogarth Press. pp. vii–162.

——. (1915). "Thoughts for the times on war and death" (*S.E.*) XIV. London: Hogarth Press. pp. 273–300.

——. (1938). *Moses and Monotheism* (*S.E.*) XXIII. London: Hogarth Press. pp. 2–137.

Lacan, J. (1976). Joyce le symptôme, Seminar XXIII. In J.-A. Miller (ed.) *Ornicar?* pp. 6–11.

Malraux, A. (2004). *Œuvres complètes* (French edn.). Bibliothèque de la Pléiade.

2

POLITICAL PHILOSOPHY IN FREUD

The death drive and the critical faculty[1]

Judith Butler

Introduction

In general, Freud is not considered to be a political philosopher, although some of his insights have been brought into philosophical positions that seek to address political issues. Sometimes political metaphors turn out to have special importance to certain views he has enunciated. On several occasions, he remarks on the dangers of nationalism, the phantasmatic character of citizenship, the problem of authority, the origins of violence and war, and the prospects for peace. At work here is an operative metaphor of the psyche as a legal system unto itself, passing judgment, asserting authority, banishing foreign elements and dealing out forms of punishment.[2] In his "Thoughts for the times on war and death," written in 1915 and in the midst of World War I, Freud reflected on the bonds that hold a community together as well as the destructive powers that break those bonds.[3] By the time he develops the death drive, first in 1920[4] and then more fully in the following decade, he becomes increasingly concerned with the destructive capacities of human beings. What he calls sadism, aggression and destructiveness come to be primary representatives of the death drive which receives its most mature formulation in *Civilization and Its Discontents* in 1930.[5] What he called an "unconquerable part of human nature" in *Beyond the Pleasure Principle* 10 years earlier takes on a new form as Freud develops a dualistic metaphysics, counter-posing Eros, the force that creates ever more complex human bonds, to Thanatos, the force that breaks them down. A durable political form presumes that social bonds can remain relatively in place, but how, then, do polities deal with the destructive force that Freud describes?

The effort to understand how a social bond is forged and maintained leads us to Freud's view that it is Eros that compels us to create and sustain human bonds, even to elaborate increasingly complex human bonds. Thus, according to that view, polities that depend on the possibility of continuing and expanding increasingly complex human ties may be said to rely upon Eros in some way. If they presume that people will be oriented towards maintaining and cultivating such ties, then those polities – and the political philosophies by which they are conceptually grasped – presume the workability of those bonds and must, as a result, anticipate their breakability as well. In his reflections on war, for instance, the breakability of those bonds becomes for Freud a pressing matter for reflection.

The death drive

Until 1920, Freud maintained that psychic life was governed by pleasure, sexuality or libido, and it was only when he encountered forms of war neurosis that he began to consider that there were symptoms characterized by compulsive repetition that could not be explained by wish-fulfillment or a drive towards gratification. So it was in the wake of war that Freud began to formulate the death drive, prompted as well by his consideration of forms of destructiveness with a repetitive quality that seemed distinct from all erotic satisfaction (what he will later refer to as "non-erotic aggressivity" in *Civilization and Its Discontents* (1930, p. 120)). In the first formulation of the death drive in *Beyond the Pleasure Principle*, Freud sought to find an explanation for forms of repetitive behavior that did not appear to be guided by satisfaction. He had encountered patients suffering from war neurosis who relived traumatic scenes of violence and loss in ways that bore no clear resemblance to forms of repetition linked with libido and wish-fulfillment. There appeared to be no satisfaction linked to this kind of uncontrollable repetition of suffering, progressively deteriorating the condition of the patient. At this stage, Freud developed the first version of the death drive according to which the organism seeks a return to its primary inorganic state, a state relieved of all excitation. Indeed, every human organism seeks to return to this origin such that the trajectory of a life turns out to be no more than a "circuitous route towards death."[6] As much as there is something in humans that seeks to fulfill wishes and to preserve its own organic life, there is also something that operates to the side of wish-fulfillment, seeking to negate the organic conditions of life, whether that life belongs to another or to oneself.

At this point Freud effectively calls into question one of the key tenets of classical liberal political philosophy – namely, that the primacy of self-preservation functions as a presupposition in the formation of social groups and forms of government. If one were to argue in a Hobbesian vein that self-interest or self-preservation leads humans into war, one would be neglecting that very dimension of destructiveness that Freud seeks to foreground, one that potentially works against both self-interest and self-preservation. Freud's point is important since it would seem that political forms depend upon the preservation of social bonds, so if something works to destroy those bonds, it works to undermine the basis of political community as well. The preservation of social bonds presumes that beings not only seek to preserve themselves as individuals, but as a social creature for whom preservation depends upon ongoing social relations. The workability of this claim presumes, however, that self-preservation is bound up with social relations – that is, the "self" who is preserved is defined in fundamental ways by its social relations and not only or primarily as an individual.

If a being whose primary aim is self-preservation has to live with others who have the same primary aim, then how do they seek to (a) secure the preservation of each other's lives and (b) develop forms of concern for society as a whole? One answer to that dilemma has been to show that society itself secures self-preservation, and so fulfills that primary aim of human life. What difference does it make that Freud now posits another tendency within the human psyche that seeks to return it to a time before the individuated life of the human organism? If self-destruction is equally powerful as self-preservation, what implications does that have for the political forms in which people live? His reflections on destruction focus on the possibility of the destruction of other lives, especially under conditions of war, in which the technology of weaponry amplifies the powers of human destructiveness. Those who suffered war neurosis were living out the psychic consequences of war, but they also became the occasion for Freud to consider how destruction works not only against others, but against oneself. War neurosis continues the suffering of war in the form of traumatic symptoms characterized by repetition. This form of repetition serves no wish-fulfillment, progressively deteriorating the condition of the patient with no end in sight. Freud identifies this as the repetitive character of destruction. In the patient, it eventuates in social isolation; more broadly considered, it not only serves to weaken the social bonds that hold societies together, but also to deteriorate the human organism, taking form as a self-destruction that can culminate in suicide. Libido or sexuality has a reduced or vanishing role in this form of destruction, and the social bonds without which political life proves impossible are shredded in its midst. Of course, there are communities and bonds of solidarity that are formed under conditions of war, apparently vitalized by shared – transitively communicated – aims of destruction. We see this across the political spectrum, social bonds formed in resistance or in opposition, taking up arms to achieve their goals. The more general point, however, is that certain conditions of destruction erode and potentially destroy even those forms of social relations, since trauma disconnects a subject from itself and from the other. When this happens on a large scale, the social basis of political life is imperilled; repair and renewal are indefinitely suspended.

Towards the end of *Beyond the Pleasure Principle*, Freud asserts that every human organism in some sense seeks its own death, and that this tendency cannot be derived from the sexual drives. The evidence for the death drive, he argues, can be found within sexual sadism and, more generally, within the phenomenon of sadomasochism.[7] Although the sexualization of the death drive can subordinate its destructiveness to what Freud regards as the non-destructive aims of sexuality, the death drive can come to predominate – a situation that would be illustrated clearly with sexual violence. Both self-destruction and the destruction of the other are potentially at work within sadomasochism, suggesting for Freud that a drive separate from the sexual drive can nevertheless operate through it. Fugitive and opportunistic, the death drive seizes upon sexual desire without properly or explicitly making itself known. A sexual relation that begins with the desire to join together becomes interrupted by myriad forms of self-destruction that seem manifestly counter to the stated aims of the lovers. The disconcerting quality of acts that are clearly self-destructive or that destroy the bonds that one wants most to keep is but one ordinary form of wreckage by which the death drive makes itself known in sexual life.

In *Civilization and Its Discontents* (1930), another text concerned with the potentially destructive effects of war, sadism is once again introduced as the "representative" of the death drive, but in this late work the death drive is more explicitly linked with the concepts of aggression and destructiveness. These latter are no longer understood as operating exclusively in the context of sexual sadomasochism for, as Freud remarks, "we can no longer overlook the ubiquity of non-erotic aggressivity and destructiveness."[8] Freud is registering the escalation of bellicosity and nationalism across Europe as well as the strengthening of anti-Semitism. These forms of aggression are not linked with pleasure or with the satisfactions that belong to pleasure: "This aggressive instinct [drive] is the derivative and the main representative of the death instinct [drive] which we have found alongside of Eros and which shares world-dominion with it."[9] Even though what he now calls "Eros" and "Thanatos" do not usually occur separately, they nevertheless have contrary aims: Eros seeks to combine or synthesize separate units within society, bringing individuals together into groups, but also bringing groups together in the service of larger social and political forms. Thanatos drives those same units apart, and even drives each unit apart from itself. So in the very action that seeks to establish and build a social bond, a counter-tendency exists that just as readily seeks to take it apart – i.e., I love you; I hate you; I cannot live without you; I will die if I continue to live with you.

Freud has two different ways of approaching this problem in relation to love. On one hand, he insists throughout his work on the constitutive ambivalence in all love relations. This becomes clear in his chapter on "emotional ambivalence" in *Totem and Taboo*, but also in "Mourning and Melancholia," where the loss of the loved one is coupled with aggression.[10] On that model, love is itself ambivalent.[11] On the other hand, "love" is another name for "Eros" and names only one pole in the polarity of emotional ambivalence. There is love and there is hate. So either love names the ambivalent constellation of love and hate, or it is but one pole of that bipolar structure. Freud's own position seems itself to be ambivalent, perhaps rhetorically yielding further proof of his claim. Indeed, the paradoxical formulation is never fully resolved in his writings, remaining fecund throughout. It surfaces symptomatically in the late work: love is that which binds one person to another, but love, by virtue of its inherent ambivalence, contains the potential to destroy social bonds. Or, at least, if it is not love that destroys those bonds, there is a destructive force that is in love or attaches itself to love, that moves human creatures towards destruction and self-destruction, including the destruction of that which they most love.

The fact that Freud's mind remains unsettled on the question of whether love contains or opposes this destructiveness is a sign of a problem that continues as he attempts to think not only about intimate relations of love but the psychology of the mass and its destructive potential. Is the destructive capacity to be found within the bonds that hold such groups together – a sort of destructive tie, or is it rather a power that "cuts all the common bonds" – an anti-social impetus that tears at social relations?

What happens in groups, large crowds, or what Freud calls "masses," such that destructive aims can take hold as they do? Although Freud does not lead with this question in *Group Psychology and the Analysis of the Ego* (1922) it surfaces insistently throughout the course of that text, more aptly translated as *Mass Psychology and the Analysis of the Ego*.[12] Freud notes in that text the tendency for individuals to yield their judgment or "critical faculty" in the midst of groups, especially those compelled by a leader, and engaged in forms of mutual excitation by the prospect of violence.

The critical faculty and the mass

In his discussion of Gustave Le Bon's *The Crowd: A Study of the Popular Mind*, Freud seeks to take account of what Le Bon calls "the invincible power which allows [the individual] to yield to instincts which, had he been alone, he would perforce have kept under restraint."[13] The individual is "less disposed to check himself" in an anonymous crowd.[14] Freud is sceptical about whether individuals suddenly acquire new attributes in the midst of a crowd or whether, as seems more likely, what emerges are unconscious impulses that are suddenly less restrained by conscience or a sense of responsibility in the context of the group. In 1922 at least, his view is that conscience is a matter of "social anxiety" – wondering what others think and feeling constrained by their judgments. A crowd that encourages its members not to worry about what others think will be relieved of inhibition and social anxiety alike.

Freud finds two interconnected descriptive terms in Le Bon quite useful for understanding what crowds do under conditions of disinhibition. The first is contagion, where the suggestion is made that contagious affect within crowds belong: to an "hypnotic order" in which the individual sacrifices his own interests for those of the collective.[15] The second point is related, and it has to do with suggestibility, understood as the subjective condition of yielding to an external impression. Whereas Le Bon relies on terms like "magnetic attraction" to explain this phenomenon, Freud remarks that those who are under the influence of suggestion – and so still within an extended region of hypnosis – undertake actions with what Le Bon calls an "irresistible impetuosity" that is increased in the midst of crowds.[16] So contagion is the central phenomenon, and suggestibility takes a more heightened form when coupled with contagion. But perhaps most importantly, the crowd is governed by unconscious motives, and those are brought forth by grand gestures: powerful images, exaggerations and repetitions –

"saying the same thing again and again."[17] The crowd expects a tendency towards violence. In Freud's words, "it wants to be ruled and oppressed." Precisely because Le Bon does not acknowledge any repressed content breaking out in violence, it becomes Freud's task to rethink how and why disinhibition is related to the unconscious. Freud disputes the notion that there might be hereditary grounds for the desire for an authority to which a crowd might submit. In this way, herds of animals and groups of people behave the same way: "a group is an obedient herd."[18] Yet Freud makes clear that the mass can find a leader only if the leader himself is "held in fascination by a strong faith (in an idea)" – only by exhibiting and communicating his own powerful belief can the leader compel the powerful belief of the mass.[19] Freud writes of the leader, "he must possess a strong and imposing will, which, the group, which has no will of its own, can accept from him."[20] In effect, his will becomes their ether – the pure essence that the gods breathe. What Freud does not immediately say, but adds later, is that as much as the mass accepts his will, the leader's will is strengthened by their belief.[21] The result of attributing such powers to a leader is the effect of "prestige" and what Freud describes as the paralysis of "the critical faculty."[22] Later, he remarks that within a crowd, perceiving someone else with heightened affect evokes a sympathetic response – a form of primitive sympathy – that induces in the perceived person the same affect. This compulsion becomes stronger the more heightened the affect, and the affect heightens precisely through the sorts of contagious communications that take place in crowds. Relying on the work of William McDougall on the group mind,[23] Freud remarks that "the most remarkable and also the most important result of the formation of a group is the 'exaltation or intensification of emotion produced in every member of it'" – the result of a "direct induction" of heightened affect.[24] As a consequence, "the individual loses his power of criticism."[25] Then again, Freud reiterates McDougall: "the collective lowering of intellectual ability is avoided by withdrawing the performance of intellectual tasks from the group and reserving them for individual members of it." And then Freud refines the formulation: qualities are conferred upon the mass "which were characteristic of the individual" and those qualities are the very ones that have been effaced by the formation of the mass.

So Freud tells us that to some degree the formation of a mass makes us stupid or, rather, people congregating lose their critical faculty in concert because they have relegated the task of thought to someone else, or perhaps to no one, letting the mass replace the individual, savoring self-loss over the travails of individuation.[26] Further, the heightening of affect correlates with the "collective inhibition of intellectual functioning."[27] So though we think of mass formation as providing the condition for letting inhibitions go, the mass actually strengthens one sort of inhibition, the inhibition of critical thought. Where the inhibition of anti-social impulse once reigned, the inhibition of thought now prevails, loosening the inhibition on anti-social impulse. We have not, it seems, overcome inhibition – as seemed to be the promise – but only shifted its locus and, as it takes form as disinhibition, its operation is inverted.

Freud's view is that critical thought has the power to inhibit forms of affective excitation and, inversely, heightened affect can inhibit the critical faculty. So the task that emerges for Freud is less to strengthen the powers of inhibition in general than to strengthen the inhibiting power of the critical faculty. When that heightened affect becomes a form of group cruelty, is the obligatory task to strengthen the social bonds apparently supported by love (strengthening Eros against its adversary, Thanatos) or to strengthen and sharpen the critical agency that will, in *The Ego and the Id* (1923), come to be identified with the super-ego? Here Freud is interested not only in diagnosing forms of crowd conduct that portend destruction, but also finding and strengthening whatever capacities humans have to counter such formations. Whereas love is sometimes identified as the counter-force to destruction, at other times it seems it is this "critical faculty" that is most important. In *Group Psychology*, the "critical faculty" describes various forms of deliberation and reflection, but the next year it takes on a new meaning and is associated with the super-ego, a form of cruelty unleashed upon the ego. Eventually, the super-ego will become identified as "a pure culture of the death drive" at which point the way to counter destruction is through deliberate forms of self-restraint – i.e. directing destructiveness against one's own destructive impulse (i.e. self-restraint is a deliberate and reflexive form of destructiveness directed against the externalization of destructive aims).[28] In other words, the check against unleashing destructive impulse which earlier could be described as an inhibition is set up as a psychic mechanism once Freud introduces the super-ego. The task of the super-ego is to direct its destructive power against its destructive impulses. The problem with this solution, of course, is that an unbridled operation of the super-ego can lead to suicide, converting the destruction of the other into the destruction of the self. On one hand, the "critical faculty" seems attentive to the consequences of action, monitoring forms of expression and action to prevent injurious consequences. On the other hand, as an expression of the death drive, its aim is potentially destructive of the ego itself. A moderate form of self-checking can explode into unrestrained suicidal self-beratement, but only if the death drive itself remains unchecked. Paradoxically, this means that the critical agency upon which one relies to check destructive impulse can become the instrument of destructive impulse, imperilling the life of the ego itself. Thus, the self-preserving tendencies of Eros have to be applied to the death drive as a check on its destructive operation. If the super-ego works destruction against the ego to inhibit its destructive expression, it still traffics in destruction, but the imperiled object is no longer the other or the world, but the ego itself. Thus, the critical faculty is of limited use in checking destruction, since it cannot check the destruction that operates through its super-egoic form. For that, a countervailing force is needed, one that pursues self-preservation and, more generally, the preservation of life. Is that force to be called love, or is it mania? Does it involve disidentification, or the adoption of a neurotic position that establishes a critical distance from the sadistic exhilarations that run through society?

Of course, the task of checking uninhibited forms of destructiveness is not an easy one, mired as it is in certain constitutive paradoxes. If the super-ego were sufficient, we would have no problem, but once the super-ego is understood as potentially destructive as well, there seems to be no way out of the circle of destructiveness. What difference does it make if we return to the mass psychology to pose this question? For the problem is not how the super-ego relates to impulse (id) or the ego (reality principle), but what happens within groups: What are the perils and the promises? How does a return to this focus resituate our discussion of destructiveness?

Freud probes these questions in earnest in *Group Psychology and the Analysis of the Ego* a year or so before the development of the theory of the super-ego: What is the mechanism by which the disinhibition of cruelty takes place? How do we account for its workings? And what, for instance, does disinhibition have to do with identification, the process by which group identities are formed? When we say that a wave of feeling passes through a crowd, what do we mean? Or when certain kinds of passions are *unleashed* in a crowd that would otherwise remain unexpressed, how do we account for that expression? Does "unleashing" mean that a desire was always there, but simply held in check? Or is "unleashing" always structured, and so giving form to the desire or rage as it emerges? If we say that an elected official has licensed a new wave of misogyny, or that he has made widespread racism permissible, what sort of agency do we attribute to him? Was it there all along, or has he brought it into being? Or was it there in certain forms and now his speech and action give it new forms? In either case, impulse is structured, either by the power by which it is repressed that designates and shapes it in some way, or by that power by which it is "liberated" which endows it with specific meaning in relation to the prior repression. If we were simply to accept a hydraulic model or one that holds that a quantity of "energy" is released when inhibition is lifted, then the impulse is the same whether it is inhibited or expressed. But if it matters through what means the inhibition has been enforced, and that means crafts the content of the repressed, then the emergence of the formerly inhibited impulse does not simply push aside the inhibiting force; rather, it wages an orchestrated attack on that form of power, debunking its reasons, its legitimacy, it claims. The impulse that emerges is thus worked over with interpretations and no raw energy, defined in relation to prohibition and license. It has actively contested the moral and political claims that have informed and supported the inhibition; it has worked assiduously against the critical faculty – not just moral judgments and political evaluations, but the general character of reflective thought that make both possible. The impulse seeks to disperse and nullify moral self-restrictions, the basis for what Freud comes to call the super-ego itself. It may seem that against such a challenge to the super-ego, the task is to shore up moral restrictions, especially those that the self imposes on itself. But once it becomes clear that the super-ego is itself a potential force of destruction, the matter becomes more complex.

Freud's reflections can tell us something about what a common or shared use of the critical faculty looks like, or what it entails, what its fault lines are, and why groups and political formations can persist only when a moderating version of the critical faculty stays alive, one that can check both the external expression of destructive aims and its self-destructive internalization. The point is not to model society on the ego, but to ask about the specific social forms that destruction can take and what implications they have for shared political life. On one hand, Freud gives us a psychological explanation of the conditions under which groups can survive without destroying others or themselves. On the other hand, a political principle is developed that shows the importance of mass psychology for political philosophy – namely, that for societies that wish to organize themselves on the basis of a principled opposition to cruelty – that is, to war or to the death penalty – there first has to be a mindfulness of the destructive potential that inheres in all group formations, and then a shared sense of the form and power of a critical faculty, a form of judgment, that knows how and when to check that destructiveness and that has the power to do so. Such judgment is crucial to the operation of politics, and one task of political theory is to establish the conditions of its possible exercise.[29]

Notes

1. This chapter constitutes part of the chapter "Political philosophy in Freud: War, destruction, and the critical faculty" in *The Oxford Handbook on Psychoanalysis and Philosophy*, edited by Michael Lacewing et al., Oxford: Oxford University Press, 2019. In press at time of writing.
2. Sigmund Freud, *The Ego and the Id*, 1923, in *The Standard Edition of the Complete Psychological Works of Sigmund Freud* (subsequently abbreviated as *S.E.*, 1956–1974), trans. and ed. James Strachey et al., London: The Hogarth Press and the Institute of Psychoanalysis, vol. XIX, 1–59.
3. Freud, "Thoughts for the times on war and death," 1915, *S.E.* XIV, 273–300.
4. Freud, *Beyond the Pleasure Principle*, 1920, *S.E.* XVIII.
5. Freud, *Civilization and Its Discontents*, 1930, *S.E.* XXI.
6. In *Beyond the Pleasure Principle*, Freud describes the "circuitous route to death" that a life takes, governed in fugitive fashion by a drive that seeks to return to an inorganic condition (38).
7. Freud's theorization of sadomasochism seeks to explain the phenomenon through recourse to the theory of libido both in "Instincts and their vicissitudes" (1915) but become revised in light of the death drive in *Beyond the Pleasure Principle* (1920) and "The Economic Problem of Masochism" in 1923.
8. Freud, *Civilization and Its Discontents*, *S.E.* XXI, 120.
9. Ibid., 122.
10. Freud, "Mourning and Melancholia," 1917, *S.E.* XIV, 248–252.
11. Ibid., 250.
12. Freud, *Group Psychology and the Analysis of the Ego*, *S.E.* XVIII, 67–145. In German, it is not group psychology, but "mass psychology" (*Massenpsychologie*) which carries a sense of much larger crowds, drawing on Le Bon's analysis of the crowd. In the Penguin edition published in 2004 and translated by J. A. Underwood, the text is appropriately entitled *Mass Psychology and the Analysis of the "I."*
13. Gustave Le Bon, *The Crowd: A Study of the Popular Mind*, New York: Dover, 2002, 15, originally published in 1895 as *Psychologie des foules*.

14. Ibid.
15. Freud, *Group Psychology and the Analysis of the Ego, S.E.* XVIII, 75.
16. Ibid., 76.
17. Ibid., 78.
18. Ibid., 81.
19. Ibid.
20. Ibid.
21. See, for instance, France Kafka's "Josephine the singer, or the mouse folk," trans. Willa and Edwin Muir, in *Complete Stories*, ed. Nahum Glatzer, New York: Schocken Books, 1971, 386–403, for an account of how the leader – a singer – is inflated by the people, idealized in impossible terms, because they depend on her for a sense of their national unity and belonging. In the end, she is weak and barely speaks or sings, but the mechanism of their idealization stays intact, and it appears that the people (the mouse folk) are the ones with the idealizing power to sustain their leader. In the end, transience takes over, and the entire history is ushered into oblivion.
22. Freud, *Group Psychology and the Analysis of the Ego, S.E.* XVIII, 81.
23. William McDougall, *The Group Mind*, Cambridge: Cambridge University Press, 2015, originally published in 1920.
24. Freud, *Group Psychology and the Analysis of the Ego, S.E.* XVIII, 84.
25. Ibid.
26. Ibid., 78.
27. Ibid., 82.
28. Freud, *The Ego and the Id, S.E.* XIX, 53, translation modified.
29. See Linda Zerilli, *A Democratic Theory of Judgment*, Chicago: University of Chicago Press, 2016.

References

Alford, C. F. (1994). *Psychoanalysis in Political Theory: Group Psychology and Political Theory.* New Haven, CT: Yale University Press.

Balibar, E. (2017). The invention of the superego: Freud and Kelsen, 1922. In *Citizen Subject: Foundations for Philosophical Anthropology.* Translated by S. Miller. New York: Fordham University Press.

Bottici, C. and Kuehner, A. (2012). Between psychoanalysis and political philosophy: towards a critical theory of political myth. *Critical Horizons*, 13(1): 101–121.

Brown, W. (2001). The desire to be punished: Freud's "a child is being beaten". In *Politics Out of History.* Princeton, NJ: Princeton University Press.

Freud, S. (1913). Totem and taboo. *(S.E.)* XIII. London: Hogarth Press. pp. vii–162.

——. (1915). *Thoughts for the times on war and death* (*S.E.*) XIV. London: Hogarth Press. pp. 273–300.

——. (1917). *Mourning and Melancholia (S.E.)* XIV. London: Hogarth Press. pp. 248–252.

——. (1920). *Beyond the Pleasure Principle (S.E.)* XVIII. London: Hogarth Press. pp. 1–64.

——. (1921). *Group Psychology and the Analysis of the Ego (S.E.)* XVIII. London: Hogarth Press. pp. 67–145.

——. (1923). *The Ego and the Id (S.E.)* XIX. London: Hogarth Press. pp. 1–66.

——. (1930). *Civilization and Its Discontents (S.E.)* XXI. London: Hogarth Press. pp. 59–145.

Frosh, S. (1999). *The Politics of Psychoanalysis: An Introduction to Freudian and Post-Freudian Theory.* London: Palgrave.

Gerson, G. (2004). Object relations psychoanalysis as political theory. *Political Psychology*, 25(5): 769–794.

Lear, J. (1998). *Open-Minded: Working Out the Logic of the Soul.* Cambridge, MA: Harvard University Press.

Le Bon, G. (1895/2002). *The Crowd: A Study of the Popular Mind.* New York: Dover (originally published in 1895 as *Psychologie des foules*).

Luxon, N. (2013). *Crisis of Authority: Politics, Trust, and Truth-Telling in Freud and Foucault.* Cambridge: Cambridge University Press.

McDougall, W. (1920/2015). *The Group Mind.* Cambridge: Cambridge University Press.

Pitkin, H. (1999). *Fortune Is a Woman: Gender and Politics in the Thought of Niccolo Machiavelli.* Chicago: University of Chicago Press.

Reich, W. (1933/1970). *The Mass Psychology of Fascism.* New York: Farrar, Strauss & Giroux.

Rogin, M. (1975). *Fathers and Children: Andrew Jackson and the Subjugation of the American Indian.* New York: Knopf.

——. (1988). *Ronald Reagan, the Movie: And Other Episodes in Political Demonology.* Berkeley, CA: University of California Press.

Roazen, P. (1999). *Freud: Political and Social Thought.* Piscataway, NJ: Transaction Publishers.

——. (2000). *Political Theory and the Psychology of the Unconscious: Freud, J. S. Mill, Nietzsche, Dostoevsky, Fromm, Bettelheim and Erikson.* London: Open Gate Press.

Rose, J. (1993). *Why War? Psychoanalysis, Politics, and the Return to Melanie Klein.* London: Blackwell.

——. (2004). Introduction. In *Freud, Mass Psychology and Other Writings.* London: Penguin.

——. (2007). *The Last Resistance.* London: Verso.

Rosen, A. (2007). On the fate of psychoanalysis and political theory. *Psychoanalytic Quarterly*, 76(3): 943–980.

Rubenstein, D. (2008). *This Is Not a President: Sense, Nonsense, and the American Political Imaginary.* New York: New York University Press.

Wolfenstein, E. (1993). *Psychoanalytic-Marxism: Groundwork.* New York: Guilford Press.

Wolin, S. (1960/2004). Liberalism and the decline of political philosophy. In *Politics and Vision.* Princeton, NJ: Princeton University Press.

Yanay, N. (2014). *The Ideology of Hatred: On the Psychic Life of Discourse.* New York: Fordham University Press.

Zaretsky, E. (2015). *Political Freud: A History.* New York: Columbia University Press.

Zerilli, L. (2016). *A Democratic Theory of Judgment.* Chicago: University of Chicago Press.

3

THE END(S) OF VIOLENCE[1]

Juliet Flower MacCannell

Freud's most elaborate discussion of violence came in response to Albert Einstein's urgent plea for an answer to *war*. Einstein begged Freud to find some means of refashioning human beings so they would no longer resort to violence: Einstein asked, "Is it possible to control man's mental evolution so as to make him proof against the psychoses of hate and destructiveness?" (*S.E.* XXII, p. 201).

In his answer, "Why War?" (1931), Freud resisted Einstein's eloquent entreaties. Instead, he insistently moved the question from the level of *individual psychology* to that of the *human social order*, with its ideals of law and justice that were transmutations of a foundational, originary violence.[2] While the "destructive instincts [drives] are at work in every living creature and *striving to bring it to ruin* and reduce life to its original condition of inanimate matter," (p. 211) Freud says that their only strong counter is the urge to *unite and preserve* – a sentiment which, he notes, is the elementary desire of any social body, any *community*. Indeed, it is in the *social order* where the primordial struggle between the two drives – destructive death drive and preservative or erotic drive – is continuously played out. Questions of *war* and *violence* can thus only really be addressed through the evolution of the ethics and aesthetics of the *social group*.[3]

The community is, according to Freud, a compromised form, whose desire to persist and unify its people depends on *laws* that themselves ultimately rest upon the threat (or actuality) of a "compelling use of violence" (p. 208) to make its members comply with them.[4] Law developed from violence and in fact, Freud argues, the law represents the "*might* of the community." The law's *symbolic* authority rests on the potentially *real* power to implement it by violent means.

Freud explains that human "hordes" were initiated through brute force, by virtue of the "muscular superiority" of a single individual whose greater strength granted him power over those weaker than he. He ruled by means of the violent exercise of his power that made others submit to him. Eventually, however, his weaker subjects came to the realization that they could overpower him if they were to join together and take collective action. The ability to overthrow even the strongest man by acting in concert against him thus sets up the dynamic or dialectic of ruler/subject that starts society down the path leading away from violence (*Macht*) and towards law (*Recht*). The regime of communal law seeks justice for all and peace among its members, but it yet relies upon a latent violence that can be exercised should the rulers need to enforce submission to them.

One might think this arrangement ought to guarantee a perpetually peaceful order. However, the persistence of an inequality as troubling as the primordial disparity in strength between the Ruler and the Ruled in the original horde jeopardizes this peace. The very idea that there is actually *a* "law of the community" remains just that, an unrealized *idea*, since no human community is composed of equally powerful individuals (i.e., old and young, women and the subjugated all co-exist within any given social order). Rather than the prehistoric physical disparities in strength between Ruler and Ruled, we now have disparities in equal access to protection under the law and its purported aim of justice for all. Freud continues: "The justice of the community becomes the unequal degrees of power obtaining within it; the laws are made for and by the ruling members and find little room for the rights of those in subjection" (p. 206).

Power, especially symbolic power, is rarely if ever distributed evenly throughout any social order, and thus overturning that order always remains a distinct threat. Freud points out that if a seriously inequitable situation persists for too long, a violent overthrow of the rulers will eventually occur.

Conflicts inherent in any and all social orders thus seem to preordain the eventuality, at some point, of violent confrontation, revolution or even civil war. Societies should therefore strive to meet the perennial challenges posed to the rule of law by their iniquities with an ever more equitable distribution of justice. After all, concentrating power in the hands of the few is only a covert return of the rule of *Macht* (superior power) over *Recht* (justice for all), a figurative version of (or a reversion to) the physical inequality that established the primal horde.

The alternative? In Freud's view, the only potential path forward lies in the "*cultural transformations of the members of the community*" (p. 206). He looks towards an evolutionary forceful reshaping not of each individual's mentality, à la Einstein, but towards a progress in redefining civilization's "ethical and aesthetic standards" to the point where violence and war would be "organically" reviled. It is *cultural revolution* that Freud calls for, and its transformations must apply to all members of the community, not just to an enlightened few.

Let us now consider the recent unrest in Charlottesville, Virginia, in the USA, where white supremacists, neo-Nazis and Ku Klux Klan members marched to prevent the removal of one of the icons of the American Civil War – the statue of the losing general for the South, Robert E. Lee. Such statues were not, in reality, erected in remembrance of the Civil War; most were created much later (mainly in the first two decades of the 20th century) to signify white people's return to dominance in the South and to mark the re-establishment of virtually complete control over the lives and well-being of black people via a set of "laws" that are familiarly called "Jim Crow." These laws are far from the evolved kind of law Freud saw as the pathway to quelling violence; indeed, they aggravated inequalities of access to justice and actually formalized those inequalities to the point where only one class of persons would ever find itself permanently at the very top of the social order: white people.

After one neo-Nazi in Charlottesville deliberately murdered a non-violent counter-protestor by running her down with his aptly labeled "muscle" car, injuring another 35 people as he did so, we learned that by and large the vast majority of Americans (and their culture) had indeed evolved ethically and aesthetically in the direction Freud had hoped. They turned their backs on the murderer and his fellow would-be killers, who had marched, armed to the teeth, shouting, "Jews cannot replace us!" and "Blood and Soil!" It came as a distinct relief to most Americans that significant numbers of political leaders, captains of industry and other prominent members of the community condemned these people unequivocally, as did thousands of peaceful demonstrators showing up in other cities to make clear their disdain for the neo-Confederates, Nazis and white supremacists who had boasted of their power to dominate by means of violence towards anyone antipathetic to them.

But a counter-narrative made its presence known, too, and unfortunately illustrated the degree to which Freud's hopes for progress in contesting violence through "the cultural transformation of members of the community" had by no means been universally or uniformly installed in citizens across the nation. Indeed, the president of the United States himself virtually endorsed the white supremacist and neo-Nazi groups, lending aid and comfort to their movement by declaring that there were "very fine people on both sides." He later weighed in on the aesthetic dimension as well, calling the contested statues, mostly traditional bronzes of no particular artistic merit, "so beautiful" while lamenting that so much "beauty" might soon be destroyed.

Our society's long-standing norms that delegitimized and placed these movements well outside the mainstream began to tremble. When the president's remarks drew shocked reactions, he retreated a bit, but in subsequent comments and tweets he reverted to wording generally deployed by white nationalists to recruit people into their movement.[5] Derek Black, whose father founded the white nationalist website *Stormfront* and who has since disavowed the group, discusses these recruitment tactics: "The most effective tactics for white nationalists are to associate American history with themselves and to suggest that the collective efforts to turn away from our white supremacist past are the same as abandoning American culture."[6]

The president's words caused white supremacists to assume that he supported them in their aim of forcing our society to recognize that only a single group within it deserves to be endowed with its inalienable rights: white people. Ironically enough, it is this group that is already in power, and the supposed "revolution" against the "establishment" is as false as possible, a pseudo uprising of the oppressed.

White power and neo-Nazi groups dress up their movements as engagement in a revolution of the kind designed to redress social inequalities: they portray themselves as the "victims" of the least powerful members of our society (women and people of color).[7]

Of course, the goal of these rallies is the precise reverse of a revolution calling for the rectification of serious imbalances and uneven access to justice in the social order. Instead, by calling up the imagery and slogans of the most violent time in recent history (Nazism) they are in effect declaring that no one should even try to challenge those who currently occupy the positions of supreme power in our country, and that they will stop at nothing to support and maintain those who hold political and economic dominance in the United States: white men. Theirs is a *demonstration*, then, in the literal sense: a *showing off* of their "muscular superiority" (albeit prosthetic) by parading massive firepower (for example, AK-47s) and making plainly visible their willingness to defend the supremacy of white power. Even if their rallies have inspired a minuscule opposition willing to use violence against them (the so-called "*antifa*"), what remains striking about the white supremacists is that for all their strutting demonstrations of potency and proto-violence, birthed in internet websites, they remain largely confined to the level of images, images they apparently count on to shield them from potential real violence against them. When one *antifa* walked up to white supremacist leader Richard Spencer and sucker-punched him in the nose, Spencer could hardly get over the shock.[8] He was all about flexing muscles and displaying his group's barely suppressed inclination to violence; but he was singularly unprepared for getting whacked for real.

The question must now be: Why is the framing and promoting of *images* of potential violence key for these groups? One might think it relates in a remote way to the originary violence that undergirds the law in Freud's genealogy of society, yet these neo-Nazis clearly reject the spirit of the laws in Montesquieu's sense – i.e., of *law* being what displaces and transforms rule by brute force into the pursuit of justice. Rather, it seems clear they believe that merely making a *show* of, or simply *demonstrating* a potential for violence will guarantee their success – without their actually having to go through the hard work of real revolution or commit to a long-term violent struggle.

Their job is done once they have succeeded in promoting and glorifying images of the destructive drives that Freud says inhere in all living creatures (including societies) and that strive to bring them to ruin. But their aim is not real destruction or actual ruin: they simply want to demonstrate that violence and destruction are always superior to the preservative and unifying drives by staging imaginarily the triumph of violence over law and justice. (Indeed, the lone psychotic man who took destructive drive all too literally, James Alex Fields, Jr., was already prone to vicious violence as a ninth-grader when he repeatedly attacked his own wheelchair-bound mother, long before becoming a committed neo-Nazi.)[9]

In other words, what the groups who are emerging into the light right now are engaged in is something more akin to Hegel's imaginary "struggle to the death for prestige" than an actual physical slaughter of their opponents.[10] They want cultural prestige, and they are laying claim to the right to shape and designate the winners and losers in our culture's ethics and aesthetics, the winners being those who endorse, not revile, violence. In fact, we are now at the point of demonstrating that there is no "point," no meaning to the triumph of destructive forces over preservative ones: since it is all imaginary, it behoves the makers of images simply to embellish and glorify violence and enthrone it as the cultural dominant, with the aim of ensuring that that image is never culturally dethroned, without actually destroying the whole society.

One misinterprets what is at stake here if one believes it is still just a question of the so-called "culture wars" between competing ethics and aesthetics in our civilization. This new moment is actually *issue-less* and something far more sinister, more death-like in its stillness: that of a complete reduction of all dimensions of cultural productions, cultural ethics and cultural aesthetics to a flat imaginary, on a single plane, with a single figure dominating the entire picture.[11] Such images may be animated, as in cartoons and video games, but they obviously lack the original meaning of *anima* – soul or what the Greeks called *psyche*.[12] Indeed, it is their mission to eliminate the very idea of a psyche.[13] Reducing the complexity of human life in common to mere images is yet one more of the myriad ways we seek to deny that the unconscious and its drives has any purchase on our choices and our lives.

This would explain why the current president of the United States is so invested in his own image. We might indeed say that he is the first to have truly grasped the potential of reducing complexity to 2-D with all actual serious conflicts boiled down to being a question of which (or whose) image gets the widest distribution for an audience prepared to receive the concocted image and to seek no further for what it might mean. While the US president was recently visiting the scene of massive destruction wrought in Houston, Texas, by Hurricane Harvey (and by global climate change), the only thing that animated an emotional response on his part was not the incredible human suffering taking place, but the size of the adoring crowd he drew to watch him: "I just want to say: We love you. You are special . . . What a crowd. What a turnout."[14]

We can be and are as sceptical as Freud as far as an enduring global progress in favor of justice for all and in humanity's communal embrace of values that "organically" revile violence.[15] What progress could ever be made once our social order has been reduced to being simply the site of imaginary domination? Can our society be trapped inside the mirror-stage forever and forgo the symbolization and the rich complexity of language that modulates its antagonisms?[16] What could ever contest this?

Perhaps we might take a measure of hope from our recent past. The late 1960s and 1970s were a period when the rule of Law, the structure of Western democracy and its institutions were widely and deeply challenged by multiple movements against them. There was a great deal of agitation in those years, not all of it easy to categorize as either progressive or reactionary. Jan Werner-Mueller, Professor of Politics at Princeton University, finds that in that era "there was widespread loss of belief in the capacity of societies for self-transformation through mass political actions, whether inside or outside political institutions like parliaments. Individual, rather than collective transformations mattered."[17]

The foundational assumptions of the many and varied contestatory groups or, as Daniel Cohn-Bendit called them, "*groupuscules*" (prompted largely by opposition to the Vietnam War), were the contrary of Freud's belief that the cultural transformation of members of the community must be the only real means for non-violence to ultimately prevail over our death drives. Where Freud thought that individual mental alterations were hardly the solution to war and other forms of violence, most groups agitating against the Vietnam War eschewed attempts to revolutionize the sociopolitical order and instead developed intensive techniques for persuading people, one by one, against war.[18] A popular song by the Beatles even mocked the notion of revolution, saying that you had to "change your head" instead. Protesters held tea and sympathy rallies where they subsisted on the same small portions of rice and tea a Vietnamese citizen had access to and held "die-ins" where they lay in public streets in the positions of war victims pictured in photographs. The thinking was that imaginary identification with the Asian people at war with the US would help to end that war.[19] Thus, it was back to Einstein's hope for the transformation of individuals' mentality to advance humanity's cause against man's violence towards man.

What eventually brought an end to that war were most assuredly not the individual mental transformations of many Americans into opponents of the war, since their political leaders claimed they, too, wanted the same while prosecuting it for four years longer than they promised. What ended the Vietnam War was the clear victory by one side over the other: victory by the side that had been universally deemed the less powerful, lacking the advanced weaponry and virtually unlimited financial resources of its opponent – a new kind of war, perhaps? One in which destructive, brute force did *not* dislodge a smaller community's desire to persist and preserve its unity. What decided the contest, ultimately, was not the "muscular superiority" of one over weaker others; it was the degree of communal solidarity by the Vietnamese and their willingness to band together to overthrow the stronger entity.

Sadly, moreover, the considerable energies devoted to "turning people's heads around" did not succeed in perfecting communal equality at home, either. Instead, we find the reverse – the installation of more autocratic policies and fewer protections for the less powerful members of our own society. The new right-wing mantra of "No New Taxes" was intended to be read as "no more money going to poor black and brown people."[20] Our major democratic institutions survived, though now they seemed to feel even less inclined than ever to improve the lot of the majority of their weaker constituents, although such efforts surfaced from time to time in the corridors of political power.

There was one major cultural advance in a positive direction from that time, however. Werner Mueller names it, explaining that for all the largely imaginary revolutionary fervor of the 1960s and 1970s it did produce a truly successful revolution – not in individual psychology, nor in our legal system, but in those informal "laws" that preside over our everyday quotidian conduct. It produced, he said, a transformation in our *mores* [*mœurs*],

> States and even constitutions survived all this. What changed for good, however, were *mœurs*, not least because '68 succeeded spectacularly as a form of social-cultural criticism, or in the words of the British New Left theorist Stuart Hall, "cultural rebellion."
>
> (Werner Mueller, p. 200)

His chief example is the undeniable success of *feminism* in altering our sense of where one, at least, of those unequal community members made a major move towards equality in terms of our cultural values, and not exclusively in formal legal terms. The cultural transformation was in our *mores* – our norms of behavior, our standards of interpersonal speech and dialogue – and these new norms undermined even the "soft" power of those who continued to try to oppress.

Now for the counter-revolution. Freud did not seem to anticipate the strength of resistance to and reaction against any cultural movement towards rejecting violence. There are now proliferating movements *against* the very ethical transformations that made brute violence repulsive to most of us, and *against* the cultural attainment of a measure of greater power and equality gained by society's weaker members. Open hostility to women's increase in social stature, as well as earlier gains for black people in the Civil Rights struggles, has now reached a crescendo; it boosted the election of the current president of the United States, the very nation that for a long time had been the pre-eminent example of the democratic rule of law and its advances in providing justice for all. In fact, the US did pass laws punishing violence against women, but there are currently movements pushing back against them and agitating against punishing rapists, for example. The legal reining in of violence against women hardly quashed destructive fantasies of committing it.

While a change in mores does not and cannot have "the force of law," the widespread pretence on the reactionary right is that indeed the new mores and norms are so oppressive they have to be forcefully overthrown. Not, of course, through actual revolution, but by undercutting their dominance and undermining any influence they have in our culture by labelling them as unfairly coercive "political correctness" – rather than as "ethical advancement." The effort is to portray these informal norms as cruel laws unjustly intended to rob (white) men of their inherent right to the lion's share of social and political power. They posture and threaten violence in hopes of intimidating those who would oppose them. One white supremacist preacher in Portland is now voicing the dream of violence against counter-protesters – "There will be bloodshed," he says, but adds as a fail-safe, "God's going to wipe them out one day anyway."[21]

What the marchers in Charlottesville want us to feel is the intensity of commitment to and desire to indulge in violence for its own sake. They deployed the vilest imagery of violence not for purposes of overturning the current hierarchy but to support and sustain its status quo: white people's sociopolitical dominance. Their aim is meta-conservative: to prevent any real change from that condition.

The wave that elected a president (with only a minority of votes) who is like them hostile to law, justice and democratic institutions, touted itself as a revolt against the very *mores* that urged upon us a greater social unity and rejection of the destructive drives. The revolt, they said, was against any further progress in equalizing the apportionment of power within our social order. The president's continuous emphasis on brute force (he dropped the largest non-nuclear bomb ever made – for no particular reason – on a remote region in Afghanistan just to show off its awesome power) is his made-for-TV imagery. Recall his ferocious claim that should North Korea bomb Guam he would "rain fire and fury" on it, while at the same time telling the governor of Guam that all this was good publicity for tourism to his island. The bombastic imagery resulted in no apparent military action or even military preparation for responding to North Korea's threats.

What we have now is all we need to know about the new and absolute faith in the *meaningless image* that dominates in politics today. This president clearly knows absolutely nothing about the shape of our laws and our social cohesion – though he claims we should all love each other by loving him – and his outlook on real events and potential dangers is as superficial and as flat as the stand-up life-size cardboard picture of him awarded to graduates of his (largely imaginary) university.[22]

These reactionary movements ironically turn the very thing Freud thought would end war – "cultural transformation" – into a new rationale for endless war, for promoting violence against women and minorities, and now even against "liberals." One website asks, "Can we start shooting liberals yet?" Notwithstanding such pronouncements, the "violence" of these groups is operative neither symbolically nor really: they remain firmly fixed in the realm of the imaginary. Indeed, we might call the current president of the United States the first "2-D" president, as his only concern is with the flat screen and his image on it. His hostility to books, print media, "dying magazines" and the "dying *New York Times*" is a purely function of his rejection of the dimensionality and depth required for an actual symbolic order rooted in language and in contested but shared meanings.

Let us ask why must the return to an *imaginary of violence* typify the reaction against what has been a purely cultural transformation? Our contemporary culture, with its endless stagings of violence and terror, seems rather to be moving in the opposite direction from that of ethical improvement and revulsion against violence. After all, Freud believed that aesthetic representations of violence were "sublimations" that afforded their audience a kind of catharsis for their destructive drives without consequences in reality since they partially satisfy our destructive drives. Today's intensely graphic depictions of violence, blood and maniacal serial killers, even the dull "dreamscapes" of V-R et al., point to an effort in the opposed sense – making the virtual *feel really real*, exulting in the power of the imaginary, the mere image to affect *you* and make *you* feel greater *fear* than Aristotelian *pity*. But, at the same time, they assuage your fear because the imaginary has, in itself, no power to harm you directly. I can only conclude that it is a profound horror of the real that motivates these imaginaries of violence and destruction, and that they indicate a refusal to accept the fact that an act of violence committed always affects us in the *real* – it is never anything but a traumatic encounter whose reality can only be belied by unconscious disavowal.

The seeming harmlessness of the image does not prevent its deployment by unconscious destructive drives that seek to dominate our cultural imaginary. The imaginary is no safe haven from the real of violence, and not simply because we know that the depictions of violent acts like beheadings, widely shared over the internet, have been the greatest recruiting tool for the actual murderers of ISIL and for lethal converts to the cause like Mr. Fields, Jr. These are recruits who may have long felt the forbidden urge to kill and could now attach it to an imagined social order that made murder permissible. What, after all, is the appeal of such causes as "the caliphate" and "white supremacy" except the chance for an isolated individual to offer obedience to a "greater power" that relies on violence to sustain its dominant position – dominance, that is, over the same individual who is thereby duped into accruing more power to its masters, into advertising the magnitude of their potential for violence?

The pictured violence in our media, our games, our television and film dramas may be completely fictional, but it is real in at least this one consequence: it shows a human susceptibility to domination by what Gramsci called the ruling class's hegemony over our sociopolitical order through its strategic deployment of cultural imagery. For example, we now tend to view our politics as a (non-lethal) struggle "to the death" for prestige – a Hegelian struggle for power or mastery. The endless staging of pseudo-combat among ruling powers is always virtual and an advertisement of the ruling powers' solidarity with each other. Hannah Arendt put it this way:

> Even the most despotic domination we know of, the rule of master over slaves, who always outnumbered him, did not rest on a superior means of coercion as such, but on a superior organization of power – that is, on the organized solidarity of the masters.
>
> (*On Violence*, p. 240)

These showcased conflicts are largely as pseudo as Roland Barthes's wrestling matches; they exist to illustrate that those in power can and do have real effects on their powerless subjects by deploying these images of conflict. Their real effect is to give their subjects the sense that the social world offers no options, no "out" to its seamless totality of forced choices, and that all efforts to unite with or form solidarities with other powerless subjects is futile. All that is left to their lot is to identify with the powers that be.

Once our human emotions and psychological recoil from imaginary violence are overcome, as the widespread deployment of violent images throughout our cultural productions reveals they may already be, we should be wary of the next step: remote control, robotic violence. Arendt warns: "Only the development of robot soldiers, which [. . .] could eliminate the human factor completely and conceivably permit one man with a push button to destroy whomever he pleased, could change this fundamental ascendancy of power over violence" (p. 240). "The fundamental ascendancy of power over violence" means to Arendt the deployment of imaginary violence to keep the powers that be in power. But the dreaded reversal she decries has now occurred and may make power itself violent once more: after all, the "push button" is here already in our electronic game world, but also in the existence of killer drones in use on the battlefields of Afghanistan, Syria and Iraq.

We are now at the point of a nearly complete eradication of what Arendt calls "the human factor" and what Freud might call the erotic or preservative drives: both are rendered nil when they are reduced to the flat, depthless images that deny the real of the death drive.[23] The image is the ultimate tool for playing on your emotions. The sheer acceleration of depictions of violence in all forms of media belies any hope that they are a new form of sublimation. Instead, their dramatic rise and wide proliferation tell us that it is still in the realm of culture and its productions that we must continue to try to preserve our communities and our solidarity with the drive to preserve and to unify. We need better writers, better artists, better screenwriters, better filmmakers to take on the task of making the imaginary into a new dialectic that can be put in service of the preservative drives, while fully acknowledging the danger of the destructive ones.

Notes

1. In this chapter I respond to some recent discussions in psychoanalytic discourse that link the trauma of violence to individual psychical responses to the violence of war – e.g., Michael Uebel's 2013 article in *American Imago* 69: 4, 473–505 attempts to examine "the trauma of violence" from a psychoanalytic viewpoint. He ties it to masochism as violence directed against oneself and shame. He demonstrates this in the way our culture and psychoanalytic establishment operated in the wake of World War II. In this chapter, I take up the reaction to the Vietnam War. I also respond to the recent events in Charlottesville, Virginia, and the US president's unseemly response to them.
2. Similar to Walter Benjamin's argument in "The critique of violence" (1921) where he writes of "law-creating violence and law-preserving violence."
3. I have written a great deal about the transition from a "symbolic" to an "imaginary" group in previous publications. What the symbolic order demands is an implied contract regarding meanings and the values that the social order comes to embrace. In the imaginary psychology of a group shaped around the individual ego, which has certainly come to dominate our discourse in virtually all domains (cultural, political and especially economic), the individual is indeed an integral part of a group that is simply a mirror for/of him. See my essays on "Group psychology aujourd'hui" on "Lacan's imaginary: a practical guide," and my early book *The Regime of the Brother* for my take on the insecurities of the post-Oedipal condition – insecurities that the imaginary claims to conquer.

4. Hannah Arendt would later remark: "No government exclusively based on means of violence has ever existed. Even the totalitarian ruler, whose chief instrument of rule is torture, needs a power basis – the secret police and its net of informers" (*On Violence*. New York: Barnes & Noble, 1970, p. 240).
5. Derek Black said that the president's words of praise for "the fine people on both sides" was a major turning point for recruiting more white supremacists: "[I]f you were on the fence about whether to get involved in this stuff or not, the president's O.K. is the biggest thing that's ever happened." *The New York Times*, "The Daily" transcript: interview with former white nationalist Derek Black, August 23, 2017; available at: https://nyti.ms/2vWaess (podcast).
6. A former FBI agent who worked on white nationalism says: " 'I tend to believe that these are feelings that a sizable segment of the population holds and is reluctant to express, because they know its not social [*sic*] acceptable to say these things,' he added. 'When you have someone like Donald Trump say them from a campaign podium or platform, that makes it okay to say them. That has brought out a lot of this latent racism to full expression. And that expression then influences our policy and the way we enforce the law." *Talking Points Memo*, Allegra Kirkland, "Former skinheads hear echoes of the recruitment in Trump's 'Heritage' talk" August 27, 2017; available at: http://talkingpointsmemo.com/muckraker/trump-charlottesville-heritage-same-rhetoric-white-nationalists-use-recruit
7. *The New York Times*, "The Daily" transcript: interview with former white nationalist Derek Black, August 23, 2017; available at: https://nyti.ms/2vWaess (podcast)
8. Available at: www.cnn.com/2017/01/20/politics. More recently, one neo-Nazi group planned to burn all "liberal" books in Huntington Beach, California, but after the events in Charlottesville it canceled the book burning, afraid of potential violence from those who might protest them.
9. Leaked chats by Charlottesville's white supremacists showed them before the event photographing themselves with semi-automatic weapons and discussing the right thickness of pipes for "thumping" counter-protestors, but serious engagement in virulent violence never quite materialized the way they fantasized. By a terrible coincidence when the car murder of Heather Heyer took place, a fictional story about a psychotic man who massacres a group of job-seekers by plowing into them with his stolen car began airing, Stephen King's *Mr. Mercedes*.
10. Stendhal's remarkable novel *The Red and the Black* foresaw the rise of the imaginary as key to the continuity in power of an aristocracy past its prime after the Revolution. Its means was a Gramscian hegemony over all cultural imagery. In 19th-century France, following the *Restauration* and the institution of a constitutional monarchy, the once near-total power of the nobility was restricted. It thus came to depend on the artificial inflation of its *reputation* as "men of power" to keep them in control. To maintain power they made their own culture and behavior as the model of prestige, to be admired and emulated by the masses. But in Stendhal's world, even the power of images can be lethal, as in the last clause in this quote from the book: "ou l'humilie tellement que l'autre a la sottise d'en mourir de douleur. La marche ordinaire du XIXe siècle est que, quand un être puissant et noble rencontre un homme de cœur, il le tue, l'exile, l'emprisonne ou l'humilie tellement que l'autre a la sottise d'en mourir de douleur." (Stendhal, *Le Rouge et Le Noir*, p. 148).
11. Philosopher Kwame Anthony Appiah's complaisance in this new structure may be one of the more alarming developments in academia today.
12. Descartes long ago claimed that machines were like mere animals and that however sophisticated their artificial speech might become, it would never enable them to engage in a real conversation with a human being endowed with an actual soul. The Greek word *psukhe* (psyche) means both breath and soul.
13. Recall George H. W. Bush barring anyone from "putting me on the couch."
14. "Even in visiting hurricane-ravaged Texas, Trump keeps the focus on himself," in *The Washington Post*, August 29, 2017.

15. In his "Thoughts for the time on war and death," Freud argued that some infants are able to overcome their aggressive drives even before they become socialized – i.e., before the advent of the *Nom-du-père*, as Lacan would put it. Long before Melanie Klein began theorizing the issue, Freud contrasted two factors in the control of "bad" instincts – internal and external (p. 282). The infant learns to restrain its aggressivity "from within" (p. 282) by tempering egoistic and aggressive impulses with "erotism." This is seconded in most cases by an "external factor" which is "the force exercised by upbringing" – i.e., by the rules and regulations it encounters in the social order, and which are gradually internalized. The person whose "civilization" consists mainly of the latter, of conformity to rules, has little resistance to uncivilized behavior if the rules of the game appear to change as they do under conditions of war. Then the very State that seemed to demand his constraint now indulges itself in barbaric behaviors, killing, looting, creating chaos at will. For Melanie Klein's take on this, see my essay (1991) "Mothers of necessity psychoanalysis for feminism," in *American Literary History*, 3(3), pp. 623–647.
16. Here I recommend my recent chapter on Lacan's imaginary and the politics of coming to terms with its growing dominance in post-Oedipal culture. Juliet Flower MacCannell (2015), "Lacan's imaginary: a practical guide," in S. Tomsic and A. Zevnik (eds.), *Jacques Lacan: Between Psychoanalysis and Politics*. London and New York: Routledge, pp. 72–85.
17. Werner-Mueller, J. (2013) *Contesting Democracy*. New Haven, CT: Yale University Press, p. 197.
18. Leafing through the journal *Art in America* from the years of the Vietnam War, I found virtually no allusion to its existence in any of the artworks held up for critical praise. Instead of any major artistic or cultural enterprises to resist the war, there were one-by-one-by-one formations like "Vietnam Summer" when college students spread out across America each with the goal of convincing at least one neighbor to oppose the war's continuation.
19. In response to the editor's query about how this is different from the cry of "Je suis Charlie" that erupted all over the world after the brutal assault on the staff of the humor magazine *Charlie Hebdo* in Paris, I would only say that these words expressed *solidarity* with those cultures that encourage a free press and freedom of expression – the desire to proclaim solidarity with societies that have specific laws protecting a free press and that do not acquiesce to the will of any "higher powers" or "higher authorities" such as those that the killers professed to be executing.
20. Lee Atwater, personal advisor to Presidents Reagan and George H. W. Bush, and former RNC chairman, infamously let slip not long before he died: "You start out in 1954 by saying, 'N*****, n*****, n*****'. By 1968 you can't say 'n*****' – that hurts you. Backfires. So you say stuff like forced busing, states' rights and all that stuff. You're getting so abstract now [that] you're talking about cutting taxes, and all these things you're talking about are totally economic things and a byproduct of them is [that] blacks get hurt worse than whites. And subconsciously maybe that is part of it. I'm not saying that. But I'm saying that if it is getting that abstract, and that coded, that we are doing away with the racial problem one way or the other. You follow me – because obviously sitting around saying, 'We want to cut this', is much more abstract than even the busing thing, and a hell of a lot more abstract than 'N*****, n*****'."
21. Noor Al-Sabai, "God will wipe them out: White supremacist preacher promises 'bloodshed' at future rallies," *The Raw Story*, August 31, 2017.
22. During the George W. Bush administration's adventures into Iraq, in 2003 the US Military began the "Flat Daddy" and "Flat Mommy" program, offering families of servicemen and women stationed in Iraq life-size cardboard photographs of the absent parent. Their families carried these figures with them in their daily routines, shopping, driving, going to church. Katie Zezima, "When soldiers go to war, flat daddies hold their place at home," *The New York Times*, September 30, 2006. These cardboard figures are supposed to stand in for the real loved one. These flat daddies being without depth pretend that any human being can be reduced to a handy, flat, compact, easily portable

thing, devoid of either life or death. And they show the cowardice and fear of facing death – and life – exhibited by all the current movements to "make America great again" by pretending it should never change.

23. Recently, [Russian Premier Vladimir] "Putin predicted that whichever country leads the way in AI research will come to dominate global affairs. 'Artificial intelligence is the future, not only for Russia, but for all humankind,' said Putin, reports RT. 'It comes with colossal opportunities, but also threats that are difficult to predict. Whoever becomes the leader in this sphere will become the ruler of the world'." In response, Elon Musk tweeted: "China, Russia, soon all countries with strong computer science. Competition for AI superiority at national level most likely cause of WW3 in my opinion." 2:33 am – September 4, 2017.

References

Al-Sabai, N. (2017). God will wipe them out: white supremacist preacher promises 'bloodshed' at future rallies. *The Raw Story*, August 31.

Arendt, H. (1970). *On Violence*. New York: Barnes & Noble.

Atwater, L. (2005). Deathbed confession quoted by Bob Herbert, "Impossible, Ridiculous, Repugnant." *New York Times*, October 6.

Benjamin, W. (1921/1986). The critique of violence. *Reflections: Essays, Aphorisms, Autobiographical Writings*. Translated by E. Jephcott. New York: Schocken Books. p. 280 ff.

"The Daily" Transcript: "Interview with former white nationalist Derek Black." (2017). (Podcast). *The New York Times*, August 23.

Freud, S. (1915). Thoughts for the time on war and death. *The Standard Edition of the Complete Psychological Works of Sigmund Freud (S.E.)* XIV. London: Hogarth Press. pp. 273–300.

——. (1922). *Group Psychology and the Analysis of the Ego (S.E.)* XXII. London: Hogarth Press. pp. 69–143.

——. (1932). *Why War? (S.E.)* XXII. London: Hogarth Press. pp. 199–215.

Grove, L. (2012). "HBO's bland documentary valentine to George H. W. Bush." *The Daily Beast*, June 6.

King, S. (2017). *Mr. Mercedes* (TV series).

Kirkland, A. (2017). "Former skinheads hear echoes of the recruitment in Trump's 'Heritage' talk." *Talking Points Memo*, August 27.

MacCannell, J. F. (1991a). Mothers of necessity: psychoanalysis for feminism. *American Literary History*, 3(3): 623–647.

——. (1991b). *The Regime of the Brother: After the Patriarchy*. London, New York: Routledge.

——. (2005). Group psychology aujourd'hui. *(a): The Journal of Culture and the Unconscious*, *V* (1 and 2), Editorial, pp. i–v.

——. (2015). Lacan's imaginary: a practical guide. In S. Tomsic and A. Zevnik (eds.), *Jacques Lacan: Between Psychoanalysis and Politics*. Routledge. pp. 72–85.

Stendhal. (1830/1969). *The Red and the Black*, trans. Robert M. Adams. New York, London: W. W. Norton & Company (original *Le Rouge et Le Noir*, Paris: Garnier-Flammarion (1964)).

Uebel, M. (2013). Psychoanalysis and the question of violence: from masochism to shame. *American Imago*, 69(4): 473–505.

Werner-Mueller, J. (2013). *Contesting Democracy*. New Haven, CT: Yale University Press.

Zezima, K. (2006). "When soldiers go to war, flat daddies hold their place at home." *The New York Times*, September 30.

4

THE SEX IN THEIR VIOLENCE

Eroticizing biopower

Todd McGowan

The emergence of biopower

In the 1970s, Michel Foucault notices two radical changes in the way that violence operates. Concerning the first of these changes, he claims that at the beginning of the 19th century, state violence began to function in a much more obscure and subterranean fashion. Whereas violence had hitherto appeared in dramatic spectacles, like public executions meant to make an impression on the people, in the early 1800s violence becomes more creative and less open. The domain switches from broad daylight to the obscurity of night.[1] The new century marks the emergence of a new form of violence, in which discipline comes to replace punishment as the fundamental form that violence adopts. Violence continues to be operative, but it loses the visibility that had hitherto characterized it. Though punishment would continue to exist, disciplinary mechanisms would come to predominate: surveillance of private behavior would become more important than the dissuasive quality of the public execution.

But Foucault doesn't stop there. As has become fully evident only with the publication of his lectures from the *Collège de France*, he considers a second shift to be even more troubling than the first. From disciplinary power emerges what Foucault would label biopower or security. In the regime of biopower, natural life becomes the central political category. This latest form of power subjects individuals not with the threat of violence or death but with the production of bare life. In *Means Without End*, Giorgio Agamben argues that what occurs under biopower is that

> our private biological body has become indistinguishable from our body politic, experiences that once used to be called political suddenly were confined to our biological body, and private experiences present themselves all of a sudden outside us as body politic.[2]

Biopower transforms the terrain of politics from a public realm of dispute and contestation into a biological realm that concerns itself with life and the body. The violence of biopower, for Foucault, consists in its production of bare life as a political category.

In the regime of biopower, the violence of systems of power and control work their way into the maintenance of life. Subjects no longer go on living but must monitor and preserve their vitality. They might, for instance, purchase a watch that constantly checks their heart rate and how far they walk to ensure that they are doing their utmost to extend their lives. Living becomes a task that one must perform well, akin to a job where one must earn one's pay. Political questions begin to revolve around the living body and how to keep it alive. Because of this focus on the living body, the violence of biopower is even less visible than that of disciplinary power. We can see the surveillance cameras as instruments of power, but this is much more difficult to notice with the doctor who is relieving our pain.

Foucault links the danger of this new form of violence to its expansiveness in relation to the earlier forms. Both sovereign punishment and disciplinary surveillance function within certain limits that no longer apply to biopower's efforts at securing the living body. In his lectures at the *Collège de France* in 1977 and 1978, he lays out the relation between the three forms of violence as he explains, "Sovereignty is exercised within the borders of a territory, discipline is exercised on the bodies of individuals, and security is exercised over a whole population."[3] That is, the violence of punishment seeks to secure order within defined boundaries, the violence of surveillance takes control of the individual body, and the violence of biopower constitutes and circumscribes the life of a people. Biopower represents a tectonic shift in the way that violence functions. If we continue to think about violence in terms of the classical model of punishment, Foucault contends, we will miss the dangers that this new form of violence poses.

While I accept the general trajectory of Foucault's history of how violence manifests itself, what this history fails to account for is the sexualized nature of violence, a sexualization that becomes even more pronounced, though more hidden, in the era of biopower. Foucault constructs his history of violence just before his history of sexuality, a history that emphasizes the violent construction of sexuality. Even in the first volume of his *History of Sexuality*, he grants violence a structural priority in relation to sexuality, which becomes just an effect of a violent imposition on the body. Thus, the only way to escape violence, for Foucault, is to return to the body outside the strictures of sexuality. As he famously puts it, "The rallying point for the counterattack against the deployment of sexuality ought not to be sex-desire, but bodies and pleasures."[4] As a result of Foucault's decision to return to the body in order to avoid sex and desire, he cannot see fully how contemporary biopower functions or why it is successful. This lacuna affects even Foucault's most insightful inheritors, like Giorgio Agamben and Roberto Esposito. Biopower or power over bare life works not because it occupies itself with life but because it introduces death – or sexuation – into life.

In this sense, biopower is not really biopower but rather the illusion of biopower. Biopower masks the sexualized nature of its violence. It addresses itself not to living beings but to sexed subjects and to their modes of enjoyment. By sexualizing the analysis of biopower, I argue, we can see how the idea of biopower obscures a much more traditional form of violence that continues to manifest itself.[5]

Life without sex

As Foucault's analysis has it, biopower is not sexy – at least, it doesn't present itself through the lens of any sort of eroticism. In fact, one of the mainstays of the analysis of biopower is the reduction of the sexual or the erotic to the machinations of power. This is straightforwardly announced in Giorgio Agamben's discussion of the proliferation of sadomasochism in modern society. For Agamben, this perversion only appears to be sexual. If we look at it closely and in the light of biopower, we'll see, he claims, that "sadomasochism is precisely the technique of sexuality by which the bare life of a sexual partner is brought to light."[6] Rather than corresponding to a technique of arousal, sadomasochism, for Agamben, is an act of reduction and even desexualization. It strips away the societal form of life that obscures the living body and exposes this body to the partner. Here, Agamben is not so much analyzing how sadomasochism works as providing a phenomenological description of it within biopower. The regime of biopower extols life as the only value even when it comes to questions that seem profoundly sexual.

This reduction to life is not confined to the analysis of biopower but makes up the fundamental program of a society based on biopower. The survival of the biological body becomes more important than sustaining or restraining desires. Biopower represents the contemporary ruling idea, the idea that animates our primary concerns and interests. Worries about health and survival trump all others because life has become the highest value. In the world of biopower, there is nothing worth dying for except survival itself, which is why one goes to war not to expand one's territory or to defend a certain value but in order to eliminate weapons of mass destruction or to stop an ongoing genocide. Both the peremptory war and the humanitarian intervention, despite their apparent opposition, become privileged modes of warfare within biopower because both have as their overriding aim the preservation of life.

Prohibitions, which once had their roots in the commands of authority or universal moral laws, now derive from concerns about life and health. We shouldn't smoke or drink because these activities are harmful to the health of the population, not because they are morally wrong. The nature of prohibition undergoes a revolution as its very ground changes beneath it. Prohibition doesn't disappear as a result but rather transforms into innumerable rules for living. It is in the arena of sex that this transformation becomes most apparent.

Even among conservatives, the interdiction of sex today does not occur primarily in light of a moral injunction but a bodily one. According to the prevailing conservative ethos, one should refrain from sexual contact in order to avoid potentially life-threatening disease, not because sex violates a moral code of behavior handed down by authority. A glance at the website for one of the pioneers in the virginity pledge movement makes this clear. At the site for "True Love Waits," a prominent conservative campaign for sexual abstinence, the first two justifications given for remaining a virgin until marriage are "You are 100% guaranteed that you won't get pregnant," and "It's a sure thing that you will stay STD-free!"[7] It is not until the seventh and final rationale for saving oneself that we arrive at the idea of obeying God's edicts. This slant towards biopower in "True Love Waits," which roots itself in the authority of traditional sovereignty, reflects the ubiquity of the turn from sex to life. Biopower takes the sex out of sex and turns it into a question of survival. The violence of the sexual interdiction becomes hidden beneath the organization's professed concern for the teenage body and life.

Foucault's argument about biopower is that its hiddenness in relation to earlier forms of power constitutes a greater danger. While everyone could recognize the horrific torture of Damiens the regicide as an act of violence, the violence inhering in the publication of the latest nutrition guidelines is more difficult to discern. They seem like simply a helpful tool to keep the population healthy. And yet, the violence inherent in nutrition guidelines seizes the body more profoundly than the soldiers who tear apart the body of Damiens (an act that Foucault famously recounts in the opening of *Discipline and Punish*). One can resist, at least psychically, the violence of the sovereign torturer, but even the position from which one would resist biopower falls within its auspices, as we can see with the homeopathic movement, a form of resistance to the contemporary medical regime. Homeopathy shares biopower's investment in the preservation of life as the supreme value, though it wants to preserve life by other – and even better – means.

The fundamental problem with the elevation of life into the only value is that this process ironically renders life valueless. This is the contradiction at the heart of biopower that it must struggle against and that Foucault doesn't address. Life has a value only when we submit it to a cause other than life – that of a nation, an ideal, an ethical principle or a transcendent entity. For the subject of the signifier, animal life does not suffice for engaging our desire to sustain that life. It requires something else. For Alain Badiou, the event makes our lives worth living, but one can't find events in the natural world. As he puts it, "there are no natural events, nor are there neutral events. In natural or neutral situations, there are solely *facts*."[8] We can live amid facts, but neither facts nor natural life can give us a reason to live. The transcendence of bare life occurs through sexuality, which is precisely what Foucault writes out of his analysis of violence.

Sexuality is not our manner of procreation but instead names what in the subject cannot be reduced to procreation or the perpetuation of life. It is what renders the perpetuation of life – or sometimes the sacrifice of life – worthwhile for us. Human sexuality never remains within the confines of reproduction but instead touches on all areas of our lives. This is the founding insight of psychoanalysis: sex penetrates into all aspects of our lives because it is the indication of our inability to act as a neutral being in the world. To say that we are sexed beings is to say that we are always out of joint, that we don't just want what we want.[9] In contrast to human sexuality, animal sexuality remains within its confines and produces satisfaction, but the result is that animal sexuality cannot become the basis of the formation of values. Human sexuality can give life value because it emanates through life and colonizes every aspect of human life. It transforms the human body into a subject.[10]

If we were simply biological or animal beings, we would not be sexed in the sense that Freud understands the term. We would find biological life satisfying and not invent ways of derailing or complicating it. The inability to find satisfaction in bare life militates against the possibility of a regime of pure biopower. My claim is that in order to eroticize life and make life worth living, every regime of biopower must have recourse to death. Death stands in for castration and thus serves as a psychic reminder of the body's sexualization.[11] Death reminds us that we are subjects and not just bodies. The return of death in the midst of the politics of life gives the lie to Foucault's understanding of biopower. Biopower's announced concern for the production and reproduction of life hides its unconscious reliance on death to sexualize life.

Death in the midst of life

In his lecture course entitled "*Society Must Be Defended*," Foucault recognizes that biopower's embrace of killing and death represents a theoretical problem for him. It implies that sovereign power remains active despite the emergence of the supposedly distinct biopower that marginalizes the sovereign. Foucault contrasts these two forms of power in terms of their relationship to life and death. He notes: "The right of sovereignty was the right to take life or let live. And then this new right is established: the right to make live and to let die."[12] Whereas sovereignty exerts its power through killing, biopower occupies itself with producing life and avoids producing death. And yet, what Foucault identifies as the forefront of biopower – the Nazi state – inflicts as much death as any form of sovereign power. In his final lecture of the series, Foucault explains biopower's turn to killing through the role of racism.

The admixture of biopower and racism, a synthesis which Foucault sees manifesting itself even in capitalist democracy and socialism, reactivates the sovereign right to kill amid the reign of biopower. According to Foucault, racism allows a biopolitical regime to separate the population identified with the production of life and another population that can be put to death. Racism divides the biological field in two. As the Nazi state creates a healthy German biopolitical body, at the same time it destroys Jewish life.[13] Biopower gives life to Germans and reserves death for Jews. This explanation leaves unanswered the question of why biopower requires this division and this death-making power. Foucault simply shows how it arises, not why it does, and as a result, his explanation has proven unsatisfying even to proponents of biopolitical analysis.

One such is Roberto Esposito, who attempts to derive the emergence of the politics of death more directly from the politics of life. Esposito's thesis is that the very logic of promoting and invigorating life requires ridding society of that which threatens the purity of life. For the Nazis, the Jews are bacteria, a form of degeneration that must be eliminated in order to maintain a healthy German population. Nazism kills in the name of life and for the sake of life. As Esposito puts it:

> The disease against which the Nazis fight to the death is none other than death itself. What they want to kill in the Jew and in all human types like them isn't life, but the presence in life of death: a life that is already dead because it is marked hereditarily by an original and irremediable deformation; the contagion of the German people by a part of life inhabited and oppressed by death.[14]

According to Esposito, the turn to killing is not a return to sovereign power but the natural outgrowth of biopower. The production of life necessitates taking life for the sake of its purification.

Though Esposito's explanation is more satisfying than Foucault's because it roots Nazi killing in the structure of biopower itself, it continues to share an assumption that ultimately undermines Foucault's entire analysis of biopower. Both assume the value and desirability of life in itself and fail to investigate how life becomes valuable or how it retains its value.[15] In this sense, the theorists of biopower fall for the ideology of the system that they analyse. Foucault assumes that beings naturally desire the promulgation of health and life. There is no other explanation for why individuals succumb to the lure of biopower rather than resisting it or even remaining indifferent to it. The value of life remains unexplained in his work.[16] Biopower regulates the body and life, but it must also have a mechanism for stimulating desire. Without such a mechanism, biopower would be powerless. Individuals would not invest themselves in life and would thereby become impossible to control. This is why biopower requires the constant threat of death.

If Nazism represents the ultimate manifestation of biopower with its obsession for life and health, it also gives death an unprecedented role in the structure of the social order. Participating in the deaths of the Jews constitutes one's superiority as a German, and even the Germans who silently went along with the extermination, knowing while disavowing their knowledge, could enjoy their nation through these deaths. In his attempt to understand the Nazi genocide, Jacques Lacan notes the appeal that sacrifice has for the subject. He claims, "the offering to obscure gods of an object of sacrifice is something to which few subjects can resist succumbing, as if under some monstrous spell."[17] Sacrifice proves almost irresistible because it provides the matrix through which we enjoy. The subject either enjoys its sacrifice of a little part of itself – what Lacan calls its "objet a" – or it enjoys sacrificing others. Through the act of sacrifice, we create values, like German nationality, that we can enjoy, but this enjoyment remains inextricably linked to what we have sacrificed. In other words, there is no German nation under the Third Reich without the Jew that this nation sacrificed. The Germans enjoyed their Germanity through the Jews that Germany sacrificed because violent sacrifice provides the basis for enjoyment.

Life itself or even population, in contrast, does not provide a way for us to enjoy. This represents the limit of the analysis of biopower. Even if contemporary regimes profess a concern with life, they must smuggle death and sacrifice into the equation if they are to gain adherents. If we were simply bodies suffering under biopower, we would have no reason to succumb to it. Once sacrifice and death are introduced, however, enjoyment of our subjugation to power becomes possible. The Nazi soldier can enjoy obeying orders because it requires a twofold sacrifice – both of the Jew to be killed and of any private sense of morality. Nazism produced so many followers through its erotic appeal, not through its emphasis on biology.

Contemporary erotics

Within a regime of biopower, the fundamental source of eroticization is the threat of death. The threat of death is necessary within biopower because bare life isn't sexy, while on the other hand, everything that makes us aware of the threat of death serves an eroticizing function. The encounter with death or the threat of death reminds us that we are lacking and thus desiring beings. The Jewish threat to German life and the Islamic fundamentalist threat to contemporary life both function as mechanisms for arousal. Through the attempt to eliminate these threats, life itself undergoes a transformation and ceases to be simply life. The attempt necessarily fails or acquires an infinite quality: no matter how successful the Final Solution or the War on Terror is, the threat remains, and there is more work to be done to eradicate it. Six million Jewish corpses aren't enough to end the Jewish menace. Likewise, the death of Osama bin Laden doesn't eliminate the need for the War on Terror but indicates the extent to which the threat lingers. This threat is most clearly evident in the case of terrorism, which is the ultimate form of the eroticization of life.

We typically understand terrorism as a response to frustration, a response to too much desire that has gone unreleased, rather than as an attempt to eroticize life. This is why we perpetuate the largely mythical rationale for Islamic terrorism that suicide bombing will reward the martyr with 72 virgins. The spectators of terrorism readily accept this account because it squares so perfectly with the idea that terrorists are dissatisfied subjects seeking some ultimate satisfaction. Even if most people don't consciously view the dissatisfaction of the terrorist in sexual terms, the prevalence of the account of the 72 virgins reveals that we do impute a sexual motivation to the terrorist.

This conception has almost no justification in the *Koran* or anywhere else in Islamic thought, and no thoughtful analysts of suicide bombing cite this reward as a legitimate cause. For instance, in his book on how we should understand and respond to suicide bombers, political scientist Robert Pape contends, "Many, perhaps most, suicide terrorists fit the paradigm of altruistic suicide."[18] Suicide is not done for personal reward but as a sacrifice on behalf of the community. Nonetheless, the image of unleashed desire as what the terrorist seeks extends widely, even to what is perhaps the classic cinematic account of terrorism and sexuality.

In his masterpiece *That Obscure Object of Desire* (1977), Luis Buñuel links terrorism to the deadlock of desire. Even though terrorism in the 1970s and terrorism today have marked differences, the film retains its relevance for explaining the motivations of terrorists because of the emphasis that it places on frustration. In the film, terrorist bombings occur in the background while the main plot concerns the inability of Mathieu (Fernando Rey) to access the object of his desire – not least because she is two different people. As the film shows Mathieu's frustration, it depicts several bombings that appear unrelated to his relationship with Conchita (Carole Bouquet and Ángelina Molina), but the underlying implication of the film is that a link does exist. Terrorism, as Buñuel depicts it, is the product of too much arousal and not enough fulfillment. The frustration of desire manifests itself in the explosion of the bomb, which provides a fulfillment that sexual relations cannot.[19] The further development of a society based on biopower since the film's appearance in 1977 – and the further development of terrorism – permits us to see another possible explanation.

If the implication of Buñuel's film were correct, we would expect that suicide bombers would be born of frustration – that is, they would come from the lower ranks of society; they would be outcasts; they would lack education and opportunity, and so on. But they come predominantly from the educated classes.[20] They are subjects familiar with absence of enjoyment at the heart of the Western world that they attack. By opting for suicide, the martyr brings death into a society that focuses on life and, in this way, the martyr supplies value where there is no value. The decision to turn oneself into a martyr for Islam gives one's life a value that it otherwise wouldn't have and allows one to enjoy one's remaining life and even one's death in a way that would otherwise prove impossible. The terrorist's violence represents the attempt to constitute sexuality through the introduction of death into life.

Terrorists resort to violence to constitute sexuality rather than just having sex (which seems like a simpler solution) because the problem that they confront is not sexual frustration but an absence of any sublime objects in the contemporary capitalist universe. Only violent death can assert a value that transcends the sphere of life that governs this universe. One might say that terrorists resort to violence so that sex can exist.

It is clear how the suicide bomber's act eroticizes her or his own life. In the act of sacrificing it, one gives one's life a sublime value and significance that it otherwise wouldn't have. As I plan to blow myself up, I recognize my life, through its sacrifice, as making a difference in the world. But what is less clear, though nonetheless vitally important for understanding the logic of biopower, is that the suicide bomber eroticizes all life within the society based on biopower.

Life in the world of biopower – bare life – leads to acts of terrorism because it is not worth living. It is not that the terrorist desires too much or experiences a frustrated desire, but that she or he experiences a society absent of desire. The terrorist act represents the attempt to transform bare life into something more, to sublimate bare life into a life worth living or a form of life. The key to the terrorist act lies in its random nature: we never know when or where it will occur, and this has the effect of spreading out the threat that it provides. With the violence of terrorism in the background, all life acquires a sublime value. But threats on a grand scale, like those provided by terrorism, are not enough to sustain the eroticization of life in the epoch of biopower.

Our daily reminders

In order to sustain this eroticization of life, we require continual reminders of the threat of death. These come in a wide variety of forms: in horror or suspense films at the multiplex, in health warnings about the dangers of particular foods, in news coverage of natural disasters or killing sprees, and so on. The presentation of the daily bombardment of threats always focuses on life itself and never on the political or social coordinates of the threat. Every danger appears in the form of the natural disaster: it menaces our survival, but it has no political valence. This form guarantees the eroticism of life, and this eroticism is most visible in the daily operation of the airport security line.

Much more than strip clubs or porn theaters, airport security lines have become privileged erotic sites in the world of biopower. But the eroticism there must undergo a complete disavowal. Whenever the eroticism comes to the surface, a public scandal erupts. This occurred both with the introduction of the full body scanner that enables security agents to view the naked bodies of fliers and with the enhanced pat down that involves security agents touching the genital regions of the fliers as well. In both cases, members of the public and even state legislatures rose to argue against the new measures of security. But these protests only further the disavowal of the sexualization that occurs within typical security procedures.

In the security line, an attitude of absolute seriousness prevails, which is why a prohibition on joking governs all interactions. There is no spoken hint that a process of eroticization is ongoing. And yet, in order to pass through the line, one must completely expose oneself. One must remove shoes, empty pockets, and take off jewelery. Screeners use an X-ray machine to search all luggage, purses and backpacks, and they often identify particular bags for a hand search. Selected persons receive a pat-down search, in which a security employee runs her or his hands over the body of the traveler. When they perform a pat-down body search, the security employees put on latex gloves in order to guard against any body-to-body contact, and they begin the process by asking if they may touch the traveler's body.

The pat-down search is where the sexual nature of the encounter becomes manifest. The latex gloves approximate condoms that the security personnel change for each partner, and the question about touching the body mirrors those demanded by sexual harassment regulations at certain American colleges. The typical pat-down conspicuously avoids the genital region, but it nonetheless provides for a body-to-body contact that is otherwise unheard of in the contemporary world. In the guise of seeking out a threat, the search facilitates a resexualization of the living body. It becomes something more than a living body.

The conscious goal of airport security is, of course, preventing a terrorist act on an airplane. But the unconscious aim involves reminding us that the threat of death is omnipresent and that anyone might act as the vehicle for this threat. The official ban on racial profiling in security lines actually furthers the anonymity of the threat. The security personnel don't discriminate because death doesn't discriminate. Death might come from a white grandmother just as easily as from an Arab college student. Egalitarianism helps to create an omnipresence of danger because it underlines the randomness of the danger.

This emphasis on randomness is also evident in the additional random screening of selected passengers who have already come through the security line that the TSA employed at one point after the September 11 attacks. By obtrusively screening passengers sitting in the gate area or in line to board a plane, airport security transforms the post-security area in the airport from an area in which one can feel secure to one in which one feels the potential presence of danger. These redundant searches can surprise would-be terrorists, but they also serve to surprise and stimulate otherwise unaroused travelers. By inserting additional reminders of the threat of death into our daily lives, the TSA plays a crucial role of injecting eroticism into the tedium of life under biopower.

The violence of biopower is not confined to the reduction of speaking subjects to beings of bare life. It also manifests itself in an erotics that every regime of biopower requires in order to arouse its subjects. Biopower controls individuals in hitherto unimagined ways, but the risk that it runs is that these individuals will cease to concern themselves with life and begin to desire otherwise. The threat of violent death directs their desire to life, which is why no regime of biopower can do without this more traditional form of violence, even if this threat appears to emanate from opponents of the regime, like terrorists. If the terrorists didn't exist, we would invent them.[21]

The proximity of death is the necessary obverse of a society that produces life. The role that the threat of death plays in biopower reveals the limitations of analysis that takes power as its point of departure. For Foucault, a focus on desire not only masks the workings of power but actually enacts power at the same time. But when desire drops out of the analysis, one loses the ability to understand the emergence of value. Foucault can theorize how power inserts itself into every aspect of the social process, but he necessarily leaves a lacuna around the question of what drives people to accept it. Domination becomes a function of force and mystification. In the process, it becomes impossible to contest successfully.

It is only when we theorize the role of desire – that is, the role of death and deadly violence – within biopower that its lack becomes visible.

Notes

1. As Foucault puts it in *Discipline and Punish*, "At the beginning of the nineteenth century, then, the great spectacle of physical punishment disappeared; the tortured body was avoided; the theatrical representation of pain was excluded from punishment. The age of sobriety in punishment had begun." Michel Foucault, *Discipline and Punish*, trans. Alan Sheridan (New York: Vintage, 1995), p. 14.
2. Giorgio Agamben, *Means Without Ends: Notes on Politics*, trans. Vincenzo Binetti and Cesare Casarino (Minneapolis, MN: University of Minnesota Press, 2000), pp. 138–139.
3. Michel Foucault, *Security, Territory, Population: Lectures at the Collège de France, 1977–1978*, ed. Michel Senellart, trans. Graham Burchell (New York: Picador, 2007), p. 11.
4. Michel Foucault, *The History of Sexuality, Volume I: An Introduction*, trans. Robert Hurley (New York: Vintage, 1990), p. 157.
5. For a detailed argument about biopower as an ideology, see Hilary Neroni, *The Subject of Torture: Psychoanalysis and Biopolitics in Television and Film* (New York: Columbia University Press, 2015).
6. Giorgio Agamben, *Homo Sacer: Sovereign Power and Bare Life*, trans. Daniel Heller-Roazen (Stanford, CA: Stanford University Press, 1998), p. 134.
7. Available at: www.lifeway.com/tlw/students/
8. Alain Badiou, *Being and Event*, trans. Oliver Feltham (New York: Continuum, 2005), p. 178.
9. As Slavoj Žižek notes, "sexuality strives outward and overflows the adjoining domains precisely because it cannot find satisfaction in itself, because it never attains it goal." Slavoj Žižek, *The Metastases of Enjoyment: Six Essays on Woman and Causality* (New York: Verso, 1994), p. 127.
10. Foucault's critique of sexuality and subjectivity stems from their colonial relation to the body. He views biopolitical struggle as a way of freeing the body from the constraints of sexualized subjectivity, which has been imposed on the body by a variety of regimes, including that of psychoanalysis.
11. Freud makes the connection between death and castration when discussing the development of death anxiety, which he interprets as a disguised form of castration anxiety. He notes: "the unconscious seems to contain nothing that could give any content to our concept of the annihilation of life. Castration can be pictured on the basis of the daily experience of the faeces being separated from the body or on the basis of losing the mother's breast at weaning. But nothing resembling death has ever been experienced; or if it has, as in fainting, it has left no observable traces behind. I am therefore inclined to adhere to the view that the fear of death should be regarded as analogous to the fear of castration." Sigmund Freud, *Inhibitions, Symptoms and Anxiety*, trans. Alix Strachey, in *The Standard Edition of the Complete Psychological Works of Sigmund Freud*, vol. 20 (London: Hogarth, 1959), pp. 128–129.
12. Though Foucault doesn't weigh in on the question of Heidegger's Nazism during his lecture series, his definition of Nazism as a regime of biopower would seem to let Heidegger off the hook. Though he identifies himself publicly with Nazi nationalism and with Nazi calls for a German spiritual reawakening, Heidegger never embraced the turn to biology and thus, one might suggest from Foucault's perspective, sustained a distance from what was most fundamental about Nazism.
13. Michel Foucault, *"Society Must Be Defended": Lectures at the Collège de France, 1975–1976*, trans. David Macey (New York: Picador, 2003), p. 241. Despite his theoretical debt to Foucault, Giorgio Agamben avoids this problem by insisting on the coexistence of sovereignty and biopower. According to Agamben, biopower does not arise in the wake of sovereignty but always accompanies it and results from it.

14. Roberto Esposito, *Bios: Biopolitics and Philosophy*, trans. Timothy Campbell (Minneapolis, MN: University of Minnesota Press, 2008), p. 137.
15. This assumption of the value of life itself is what separates Agamben from both Foucault and Esposito. Agamben argues that even bare life must be produced: it does not exist on its own. He claims: "There are not *first* life as a natural biological given and anomie as the state of nature, and *then* their implication in law through the state of exception. On the contrary, the very possibility of distinguishing life and law, anomie and *nomos*, coincides with their articulation in the biopolitical machine. Bare life is a product of the machine and not something that pre-exists it, just as law has no court in nature or in the divine mind." Giorgio Agamben, *State of Exception*, trans. Kevin Attell (Chicago: University of Chicago Press, 2005), pp. 87–88.
16. The other great contemporary of Foucault who is also an ontologist of life is Gilles Deleuze. Deleuze shares with Foucault a belief that we are drawn to life because life is the source of power and everything seeks power. This becomes clear in Deleuze's discussion of Spinoza where he notes, "every body extends its power as far as it can. In a sense every being, each moment, does all it can." Gilles Deleuze, *Expressionism in Philosophy: Spinoza*, trans. Martin Joughin (New York: Zone Books, 1992), p. 269.
17. Jacques Lacan, *The Four Fundamental Concepts of Psycho-Analysis*, trans. Alan Sheridan (New York: Norton, 1978), p. 275. In his seminar from the prior year, Lacan speaks more extensively on the role of sacrifice in creating desire. There, he claims, "we do not lives our lives, whoever we are, without ceaselessly offering to some unknown divinity the sacrifice of some little mutilation, valid or not, that we impose on ourselves in the field of our desires." Jacques Lacan, *Le Séminaire, livre X: L'angoisse, 1962–1963*, ed. Jacques-Alain Miller (Paris: Seuil, 2004), pp. 320–321.
18. Robert A. Pape, *Dying to Win: The Strategic Logic of Suicide Terrorism* (New York: Random House, 2005), p. 23.
19. The criminal bombers in two actions films from the 1990s, *Speed* (Jan de Bont, 1994) and *Blown Away* (Stephen Hopkins, 1994), both praise the bomb for its ability to come to completion, which they implicitly contrast with humans, who remain desiring and unfulfilled. In *Speed*, bomber Howard Payne (Dennis Hopper) upbraids bomb disposal expert Jack Traven (Keanu Reeves) for attempting to stop the bomb from fulfilling its destiny. This depiction of the criminal's defence of the bomb is firmly rooted in the traditional understanding of what motivates terrorism.
20. See Alan B. Krueger and Jitka Malečková, "Education, poverty and terrorism: Is there a causal connection?" *Journal of Economic Perspectives*, 17.4 (2003): 119–144.
21. In *Anti-Semite and Jew*, Jean-Paul Sartre says something very similar about the anti-Semite and the Jew, but his point is that the anti-Semite requires the Jew as a figure of opposition against which the anti-Semite can form a stable identity. Biopower requires the terrorist not as its constitutive enemy but as the source of absence or death within its structure. The threat of terrorism creates desiring subjects within the otherwise rampant asexuality of biopower.

References

Agamben, G. (1998). *Homo Sacer: Sovereign Power and Bare Life*. Translated by D. Heller-Roazen. Stanford, CA: Stanford University Press.

——. (2000). *Means Without Ends: Notes on Politics*. Translated by V. Binetti and C. Casarino. Minneapolis, MN: University of Minnesota Press.

——. (2005). *State of Exception*. Translated by K. Attell. Chicago: University of Chicago Press.

Badiou, A. (2005). *Being and Event*. Translated by O. Feltham. New York: Continuum.

Deleuze, G. (1992). *Expressionism in Philosophy: Spinoza*. Translated by M. Joughin. New York: Zone Books.

Esposito, R. (2008). *Bios: Biopolitics and Philosophy*. Translated by T. Campbell. Minneapolis, MN: University of Minnesota Press.

Foucault, M. (1990). *The History of Sexuality, Volume I: An Introduction*. Translated by R. Hurley. New York: Vintage.

——. (1995). *Discipline and Punish*. Translated by A. Sheridan. New York: Vintage.

——. (2003). *"Society Must Be Defended": Lectures at the Collège de France, 1975–1976*. Translated by D. Macey. New York: Picador.

——. (2007). *Security, Territory, Population: Lectures at the Collège de France, 1977–1978*. Edited by M. Senellart and Translated by G. Burchell. New York: Picador.

Freud, S. (1915/1959). *Inhibitions, Symptoms, and Anxiety. The Standard Edition of the Complete Psychological Works of Sigmund Freud (S.E.)* XX. London: Hogarth.

Krueger, A. and Malečková, J. (2003). Education, poverty, and terrorism: is there a causal connection? *Journal of Economic Perspectives*, 17(4): 119–144.

Lacan, J. (1978). *The Four Fundamental Concepts of Psycho-Analysis*. Translated by A. Sheridan. New York: Norton.

——. (2004). *Le Séminaire, livre X: L'angoisse, 1962–1963*. Edited by J.-A. Miller. Paris: Seuil.

Neroni, H. (2015). *The Subject of Torture: Psychoanalysis and Biopolitics in Television and Film*. New York: Columbia University Press.

Pape, R. (2005). *Dying to Win: The Strategic Logic of Suicide Terrorism*. New York: Random House.

True Love Waits. Available at: www.lifeway.com/tlw/students/

Žižek, S. (1994). *The Metastases of Enjoyment: Six Essays on Woman and Causality*. New York: Verso.

5

LONE WOLF TERRORISTS

Howling in the eye of the wind: the case of Adam Lanza

Manya Steinkoler

Since the Sandy Hook shootings in 2012, there have been over 300 school shootings in the USA, at an average rate of one per week (Centers for Disease Control, 2016). Since the International Federation of Psychoanalytic Societies conference in New York last year where this chapter was presented, there have been school shootings in Utah, San Francisco, Ohio, Michigan, South Carolina, Texas, Massachusetts, Los Angeles, Wisconsin and Florida. The geographic diffusion alone points to the widespread nature of this phenomenon.

Each time a shooting occurs, we hear the media injunction not to become inured, as the public complains that this is sadly, albeit uncannily, becoming our everyday reality. There was one school shooting in the USA in 1927. The next one took place in 1966. There were four in the 1970s, 6 in the 1980s, 25 in the 1990s, 48 in the first decade of the new millennium, and over 300 since 2013.

There have been many governmental studies, independently funded studies, and pieces of research by international agencies and trend-watchers, not to mention a plethora of recent books written trying to fathom the myriad causes of this exponential increase (see Boeckler et al., 2013; Langman, 2010; 2015; Lieberman, 2008; Newman, 2005). Generally, the research looks at the perpetrators and what they determine to be the environmental and social causes that create them.

The title of the panel in which my own work was presented concerned the "lone wolf terrorist," and Adam Lanza might initially fit into such a category, or the lone wolf might seem to be a way of speaking about his story. However, I wanted to question this term in order to better hear the specificity of Adam Lanza's case. First, we must wonder whether the "lone wolf terrorist" is actually alone. He is alone in terms of our neurotic understanding of "alone," but is "alone," even if he is by himself, really the correct term? We will see that he is accompanied; Adam Lanza is never alone. Whether it is voices, the demands of his mother, the constant ghost-like presence of Columbine's Dylan and Evan as ego-ideals, the near-complete attachment to the internet or the television, Adam Lanza lived in a distinctly noisy solitude.

Next, it is important to think of the act of school shooting not as "a lone wolf act of terror," but as a passage to the act that aims at inscribing the subject in the social order. Adam Lanza's mass shooting at Sandy Hook School was a way for him to exit the constant barrage of noise in his head and "make a name" for himself, to become "someone" separated from the infinity that accompanied him.

Violence as a means of obtaining social recognition is quite popular with young men today. Not only with psychotic young men, or those severely disturbed, but with men craving strong or even intransigent paternal authority, a "larger" meaning to life, and the satisfactions of group membership and participation. Donald Winnicott famously wondered what would happen to young men and their sense of masculinity in an age no longer marked by war (1946; see also Winnicott, 1964). For generations, war marked men, "proved men," giving them a place in their generation and their time. Perhaps terror and mass shooting have become the way a young man can mark himself when war is either lacking or increasingly viewed as the work of the lower classes. Winnicott reminded us that adolescence is a "violent process"; the school shooter and the teenage terrorist make sure that we do not forget it.

In "Civilization and its discontents," Freud quotes the Latin proverb attributed to Plautus, and quoted notably by Hobbes, "Homo homini lupus." It is worth wondering: is man a wolf to his neighbor today in the manner he used to be? Or have the pressures, dissolutions and failures of traditions that mark our modern moment made for pack behavior in the frozen tundra of the shimmering computer screen?

Asked differently: is school shooting an example of the Freudian malaise in civilization, or is it an attack against that very Freudian malaise? In the era of 15 minutes of Warholian fame, where imaginary ideals replace the failing family and paternal imago, and in an era where the rise of *jouissance* trumps the limiting, and certainly not profit-friendly, word, the lone terrorist and the school shooter allow us to reflect on the price of civilization before there was any profit, the one that the Freudian neurotic pays for by way of neurosis.

Freud famously replied to Einstein in the "Why war?" correspondence, opining that we would never enjoy Plato's imagined reign of philosopher kings because the great majority of people were unable to renounce the aggressive drives and would surely remain that way (Freud and Einstein, 1978). It is tempting to think of this generation of school shooters as revealing the new voice of the social order – not one of renunciation, but one that says by way of the most terrifying irony: "Just do it!" "Aim high!" or "Shoot for the stars." The war against the gap in enjoyment that speech necessitates is all around us; school shooters and terrorists are its champions.

School shootings: what we "know"

The shooters

In many of the texts on school shooting, a researcher wants to understand "who" these shooters are and what drives "them" to "kill." The aim seems commonsensical enough; the shooter is studied as a species apart. He is not socialized: even if he had been a member of the debate team, the marching band, the technology club, or the chess team prior to the shooting, now he has become a type to be "studied" and pored over like the serial killer and the terrorist. Now he is a type, and helping us spot him is big business.

The difficulty with this research is that the vast majority of people who fit all the categories do not commit any of these crimes. Most shooters are white teenagers between the ages of 13 and 21 years; a vast percentage come from families where guns are part of family life, and hunting and shooting are regular activities; nearly all school shooters have had negative educational experiences; many, but not more than half, have experienced being bullied; many have had trouble holding down jobs; many are said to have experienced "trauma"; many have moved around a lot and have had to suffer in school situations making new friends; many live in suburban America, some in rural America, and almost none in cities; many suffer from "defects" in their bodies, either real or perceived; many had generally low birth weights; many of their mothers experienced difficult pregnancies or deliveries; many are short in height or experience themselves as short; many were rejected from the military and therefore were thought by researchers to have "not been able to become men"; many have experienced sibling rivalry; many have shown a high rate of substance abuse; some have had legal trouble in the past; many are attracted to ideologies of power and role models for violence such as Nazism, Satanism and black magic; many have had specific role models and often sought peer support on websites and blogs; many have experienced job failures; and many have experienced romantic failures. Authors endlessly debate whether this or that characteristic is an important or crucial one as the instances of school shootings continue to multiply.

The causes

The second kind of research on school shooting looks for the causes, not so much in the person of the shooter, but in his environment: lax gun laws; increase in bullying; a violence-affirming environment; a general culture or climate of violence; a lack of hospitality in the classroom; the triumph of the neoliberalist security state and the converse lack of security personnel in the schools; a culture of humiliation and the converse culture of laxity or anything goes; single-parent families and latch-key kids; a domineering parent; violent video games; loner behavior; mental illness; the *jouissance* of the bystander; the rise in technology; the failure to establish viable social ties; the reduction of educators to functionaries; and individual psychopathology that has been divided into "traumatized," "psychotic" and "psychopathic" (the last being the new word for "possessed by the devil", or simply the way we describe the psychotics we don't like).

One notes with raised eyebrows that there are even those who profess that violence in schools has nothing to do with lax gun laws, and that the same violence would occur even if the strictest gun control legislation were enacted. Such gun lobby rhetoric perversely argues that gun violence is proportionate with increased gun control (see Rabin-Havt, 2016). Indeed, as is well known, after Newtown, Wayne LaPierre, the head of the National Rifle Association, announced on national TV in a news conference on December 21, 2012, in the wake of a country in mourning and a president poised to act on gun control, "The only way to stop a bad guy with a gun is a good guy with a gun." This became a major slogan for the Republican Party and has been repeated, notably, by Donald Trump, who campaigned claiming that the Orlando shooter, Omar Mateen, could have only been stopped by a "good guy with a gun." The causes of school shooting listed above have been debated by equally qualified researchers, and just as in the example of gun laxity, some deem them not to be causes at all.

The idea that we can "pick out the shooter" before he appears makes for generalized paranoia and an educational milieu of fear, which we expect will worsen under a Trump administration. School children today practice regular "lock downs" and "active shooter drills" from kindergarten through high school, and even some colleges have recently adopted the practice. Autistic and "strange" or simply shy kids are constantly sent for evaluation and testing. Not being "sufficiently socialized" and meeting the "standards" of socialization has become cause for alarm.

Unfortunately, designating "the potential shooter" is only a way to ensure that we make more of them, engaging in the very paranoia that is part of the problem to begin with, since the problem to begin with concerns the social order or what Lacan calls the Other, the treasure house of language, the current discourse that one lives in. Said differently, in a logic particular to the Other, our "discovering" the potential shooter will only continue to guarantee that he will be there.

Wouldn't know him from Adam

On December 14, 2012, in Newtown, CT, Adam Lanza, age 20, fatally shot 20 children and 6 adults. Just months before the Sandy Hook shootings, Adam Lanza had written on a website dedicated to the Fans of Columbine: "Mass murder is not amazing. What is amazing is that it doesn't happen 100,000 times a year!" We might pause at Adam's question since he asks us to consider the problem inversely: not why do people become school shooters, but why don't they?

Upon reviewing the evidence he left, the FBI stated that Adam Lanza's knowledge of mass murder was "unparalleled" in the history of crime. The boy had been at work in his bedroom for years, studying rampage shootings, and in particular school shootings. He had a 7-by-4 foot spreadsheet listing 500 mass murderers and the weapons the killers used. This research was considered to have taken years of work. Maybe nobody noticed him or knew him very well, but Adam had been preparing his day of fame for years.

How can we understand the "solution" that "becoming a mass shooter" provided Adam Lanza with? Do we psychoanalysts dare compete with the "hard scientists" who, racing to find the "cause of school shooting," are at work sequencing Adam's DNA to find what was "really wrong" with him?

Massive massacres, mass media and identification

David Cullen, whose book *Columbine* (2010) has become a classic in the field, has argued that "The media has become complicit [with the crime]; we keep score." Well, at least someone is "watching" them and knows "what they are up to." The media, that "privileged" way to keep score, unique to our time, provides a powerful and popular way to exist. For many teenage school shooters, Columbine set a template for one-upmanship. To die in the mirror, to finally become the all-powerful ideal, was the wish that a lived life could only fall short of. I quote from the confidential private session notes of a psychoanalyst colleague who has a 15-year-old boy in treatment:

> Why would I ever want to be like my father? Why would I want to be like anybody's father? Fathers can't have real power. It's better to be a teenager. Teenagers can do whatever they want. Teenagers don't have anything holding them back.

Adam Lanza was obsessed with the Columbine shootings. He regularly posted on a blog dedicated to school and rampage shootings. Research has shown that 8 out of 12 shooters directly referred to Columbine and were interested and engaged with that story, often seeing Eric and Dylan as heroes. Seung-Hui Cho, the perpetrator of the Virginia Tech shootings, in his own video recording (YouTube, 2007), referred to himself as a martyr seeking revenge for Dylan and Eric.

Aware of the "reverse autopsies" initiated after such shootings of the perpetrators by investigators, Adam Lanza prepared a photograph of himself holding guns to his own head for the FBI to find in his room. Adam Lanza knew exactly what he was doing, shooting his mother Nancy four times in her sleep before driving off to school and leaving his destroyed hard drive in plain sight next to this photo. He was preparing everything for his "appearance" on the global stage.

The imaginary identification with Eric and Dylan allowed Adam a way to exist; it gave him a peer group. But who would want to belong to such a group, and why?

The case of Adam Lanza

Daddy

In an interview in *The New Yorker*, Adam Lanza's father, Peter Lanza, a vice president at GE Financial Services, told writer Andrew Solomon that the boy would have killed him, "in a heartbeat" and wished his "mass murderer son had never been born" (Solomon, 2014). Solomon stated that Peter was "by nature not given to self-examination" and that it was "often Shelley [his second wife] who underlined the emotional ramifications of what he said."

Peter Lanza had lived with the family until Adam was 10 years old, when Peter and his wife Nancy separated. He was known as a good father who went camping with his two sons and took Adam to the shooting range regularly, until the two years before the shootings, during which time he did not see his son at all. After one such camping trip with his father, Nancy Lanza was amazed that her teenage son was able to "tie his shoes himself," an act of independence he had not been able to accomplish in the presence of his mother.

A self-avowed "workaholic," a quality his son would emulate in his monomaniacal study of violence, Peter Lanza did "not think that the children were impacted" by his "leaving the family." Further distancing himself, he stated that his son Adam was "evil." "You can't get any more evil," he said (Solomon, 2014). Mr. Lanza stated that he did "not mourn the loss of his son." Recounting that Adam shot his mother Nancy four times, he added, "once for each person in the family." It is an interesting observation and interpretation; all the people in the family have their reference in Nancy. She even gets a bullet hole for herself, a kind of maternal ground zero.

Such comments already tell us a great deal about a father who could not love his son enough to feel a loss of him and who interpellated his son as "evil," content to adopt the demonizing signifiers the social order had given him. Adam was not able to be "lost" to this father, and we can imagine that he could therefore not have been loved by him to begin with. One is tempted to hypothesize that Adam made sure that there were many fathers who did mourn the loss of their sons; indeed, he guaranteed it. The headlines after the event for days were versions of this one: "Adam Lanza is etched in the nation's collective memory" (Ziv, 2014). Adam made sure the world would remember him.

Mommy

Nancy Lanza lived according to "a live free or die" mentality, the official slogan of the state of New Hampshire she was from. In 1971, the phrase was mandated by the New Hampshire state legislature to replace the word "scenic" on all New Hampshire license plates. It was the cry of the American Revolutionary General John Stark, who declared, "Live free or die: death is not the worst of evils." This motto, one Nancy herself espoused, pegged her as a true "New Hampshire gal," one who had "a sense that guns were part of every day life" (FBI, 2014, p. 103). The Bushmaster – the name of one of the guns that Adam used that belonged to his mother – should give us pause.

Nancy Lanza was a Prepper. Preppers are people who prepare for cataclysms, apocalypses, in short, for the end of the world. Little did Nancy know how her son would provide the very apocalypse that she was waiting for. His act is a perfect example of what Genevieve Morel calls, in *La loi de la mere* (2008), the absolute subjection to the law of the mother for the psychotic subject. In the language of the FBI report compiled after the event, we read: "The mother takes care of all the shooter's needs. She did not work. She worried about what would happen to the shooter should anything happen to her" (FBI, 2014). Adam made sure she would not have to.

For all her living free, Nancy Lanza was also known to have been "ill" most of her life with what she claimed was an "autoimmune" and "genetic disorder." When investigated after the shootings, whether she actually had the multiple sclerosis she claimed to have had was disputed. She regularly complained about her "illness," though, speaking about it to her friends, and was busy trying to "overcome" it and "fight it." She had to. As a "mother of a child with special needs," she had Adam to take care of.

Adam

Adam Lanza was evaluated continually for his entire life. He was brought to psychiatrists, psychologists, doctors, social workers and a slew of evaluators, suffering problems from birth. Nancy Lanza's pregnancy was reported to have been challenging, with maternal hypoglycemia, hypotension and decreased fetal movement followed by a cesarean section. Adam had an episode of apnea during which he stopped breathing at eight days old and was admitted to the hospital.

In his pre-school years, Adam was described as an extremely active child who did not sleep well, avoided touching, and was diagnosed with early communication problems, having "made up his own language," one that only his mother could understand. The developmental assessment completed by Adam's "Birth to Three" provider indicated that Adam "fell well below expectations in social–personal development." The evaluator was unable to understand any of Adam's language, and his mother had to serve as an interpreter throughout the testing. Evaluators concluded that Adam presented with "significantly delayed development of articulation and expressive language skills." He would continually be shown to be unable to start a conversation.

In *The New Yorker* interview (Solomon, 2014), Peter said that, "Adam struggled with basic emotions" and that, as a result of the boy's difficulties, Nancy became a "stay-at-home mom after Adam was born." When Adam had to show his emotions in a school play, he took it seriously, even practicing before a mirror. Reported by his kindergarten teacher to "like rules," he was quiet during groups, sitting and hitting his head repeatedly. In the interview, Peter Lanza said that he never worried about Adam breaking any rules of any kind. Peter taught him to drive, and Adam was the most cautious driver he had ever seen.

As a child, Adam had motor difficulties, avoided eye contact, and liked rituals. At age 5, his language problems were evident to his teachers. He had an aversion to being held or touched and did not sleep through the night. At that age, Adam changed his socks 20 times a day and his mother did laundry, washing his socks,

20 times a day. The family would go through boxes of tissue daily since he would not touch a doorknob with his bare hand. Soon no one was allowed in his bedroom; he did not like Christmas trees and he would not eat his food unless it was arranged in a particular way. One wonders not so much why a child has such proclivities; one wonders in what way they are indulged so that they become facts or constants about him.

Adam was said to have suffered from "sensory processing disorder," not able to "organize" or subjugate his sensory perceptions, and was often disturbed by the world. We can see this as a consequence of what Lacan calls the failure of the paternal metaphor. In this case, stimulation cannot be pleasurable or even borne since there is no metaphoric protection from the Real. As a child, Adam once asked his father, "Why do you need friends?"

Adam was diagnosed with Asperger's syndrome early on. It was a diagnosis that Nancy Lanza would cling to, explaining everything he did by way of his "illness," including her need to be with him and stay home with him.

In fifth grade, Adam and a classmate submitted their creation "The Big Book of Granny," depicting a caregiver and a child engaging in horrific violence towards one another. The disturbing story included taxidermy, the murder of children and cannibalism. While this submission concerned his teachers and the school personnel, it did not spur a parental intervention. The depictions were far and beyond what we consider normal childhood aggression, but the work was not flagged or noticed until after the shootings.

When Adam was taken to Yale's Center for the Child at age 14, Nancy Lanza said that her son seemed as though he was being tortured in the clinical interview with the psychiatrist and that his palms were sweating. Nancy was always aware that life was hard for Adam and wanted to make her son's life as easy as possible. At the time, the evaluators recommended that Adam have extensive special education services, ongoing expert consultation, and rigorous therapeutic supports embedded into his life. All of these recommendations went unheeded by his parents. Nancy Lanza was confident she could meet the special needs of her son. The Yale evaluation specified that Adam should be "pushed to be with others" or he would lead "a deteriorating life and condition of dysfunction and isolation." One psychiatrist examiner described Adam as the "most anxious youth he had ever seen."

Nancy Lanza always wanted Adam out of school so that he would be "safe" at home. She had the idea that having him home-schooled by his parents would alleviate his anxiety. Initially, and importantly, she was denied the right to home-school Adam, by both the school and the clinical evaluators. Ever diligent and devoted, persistent Nancy would find a psychiatrist who agreed with her that Adam should be at home.

We might flag how this case underlines that "the customer is always right" ethos can interfere with, and even directly challenge, a therapeutic one. At home, Nancy would take charge of Adam's education, giving him instruction in the humanities, while Peter would instruct him in math and science. Nancy decided to "take life day by day" – and we hear the double meaning of this phrase – in order "to make Adam's life bearable," and she would define herself and her life in terms of her concern for him. One classmate of Adam's said that he remembered a birthday party where Nancy Lanza stayed the whole time and would not leave. It is worth pointing out that, under his mother's doting vigilance, Adam was severely anorectic, weighing 98 pounds as a teenager at 5 foot 8 inches tall.

Adam himself disagreed with his Asperger's diagnosis and did not want to go for individual therapy or take medication. He wrote as a teenager on an online blog: "Therapists are secular priests who assert they have some truth. If your values deviate, then you are wrong. Hence, The Rapist – mind fucking" (Langman, 2015b). Adam taught himself chemistry and generally discounted his parents' teachings. It is striking that the fact that he was able to teach himself chemistry went unnoticed by a mother so concerned about his dependence on her.

Nancy made sure she got what she wanted. Adam was first given "homebound" status in the sixth grade. This designation qualified him as "too disabled to go to school." We might pause to consider the term "homebound." While denoting being "bound" to the home, which Adam was, we should note its other more ominous connotation, given his future, of being bound for death. Adam would return to school a couple of times and for a serious stint in 10th grade, only to withdraw again. Nancy Lanza tried to supervise his education even during his returns to school. "He might have trouble with boy meets girl type of literature," she told his high-school English teacher. Nancy took her role as teacher seriously and chose the books her son read. She organized every day for him.

She "tried to eliminate all distractions," since "distractions" always caused him anxiety. Noise, for example, had always bothered Adam, so Nancy interdicted the ringing of the home doorbell. The delivery people – indeed, everyone in the neighbourhood – knew not to touch the doorbell at the Lanza's. Nancy would even refrain from cooking because, excessively sensitive to smell, cooking had always disturbed Adam. Perhaps most stunning in this list, Nancy even warned Adam's teachers of the fact that Adam was relatively "insensitive to physical pain" and she was concerned that "he might not stop doing something because it hurt."

Interestingly, Peter Lanza and Adam's older brother Ryan both testified that Adam loved school. Even Nancy said, "Adam had a goal just to get through that door [of the school building]." Nancy said that there were often lots of discussions whether Adam could "pull it together" to get to school, and he would often cry in the bathroom for 45 minutes before going to school. Peter stated that, "Adam loved the Sandy Hook school" and that as he was growing older, he told his father "how much he had liked being a little kid." Perhaps it is useful to wonder about "love" and what it means for a child to say that they love "being a little kid" as it concerns childhood psychosis and its connection to a primary maternal object, a real and too-present presence, precisely what a psychotic child would have to separate from.

At one point, Adam returned to school and experienced considerable, often overwhelming, difficulties. Nancy found a psychiatrist to evaluate Adam, allowing him once again to return home. Here is an excerpt from that evaluation:

> At this point I am strongly recommending that Adam Lanza not be compelled to attend school. He has clearly demonstrated that the experience of the school setting which has an intolerable level of noise and unpredictable elements would promote extreme anxiety and discomfort.
>
> (Office of the Child Advocate, 2014, p. 42)

It went completely undetected to the psychiatrist that the noise and that unpredictable element was Adam himself.

Staying "safely at home" did not stop a confrontation with the law. When Adam was 14, the FBI came to the Lanza house; they had discovered that the teenager was able to hack into FBI files as well as a variety of websites. His mother brushed off the visitors. Adam was "just testing himself," she told them.

After he graduated high school in 2009, Adam placed black garbage bags over his bedroom windows and communicated with his mother via email. He stopped replying to his father's emails in 2010. And his father had not seen him for two years at the time of the shooting. For several months before the shootings, Adam stopped going out altogether.

As Adam deteriorated, he was taken once more for an evaluation. This time, it was disastrous. Adam requested to the psychologist that his father be permitted to come to the sessions. He said that he wanted his father present and agreed to the sessions under those circumstances. The clinician wrote up the session, and in a letter explained her decision not to allow Adam's father in the sessions. The letter reads like a manual "how not to be a clinician." Here is an excerpt:

> The process of asking Adam Lanza to talk with me directly about what is going on is critical. I appreciate that Adam Lanza's view is that he wouldn't say anything differently if [the father] were in the room, but I think he's wrong. His judgment about how social/family dynamics work in a therapy situation is no more on target than his views regarding doorknobs and hand-washing . . . He wants to control how the treatment goes . . . While I understand that, at the same time, he can't control the treatment because his thinking is distorted and irrational. I can't agree to follow his lead!
>
> (Office of the Child Advocate, 2014, p. 54)

When Adam was interviewed by a high-school evaluator and asked to list three wishes, he answered, "Whatever was granting the wishes would not exist!" This evaluator noticed – as had everyone who had evaluated Adam before him – that Adam feared contamination by metal objects. Adam had feared metal objects since childhood. We point out that Adam grew up in a house with guns. The irony of having a childhood allergy to "metal" and killing 26 people with his mother's guns is one that even the greatest poets would find hard to fathom. Moreover, no one bothered to read the "Met AL" (Adam Lanza's initials) in the word "Metal."

Adam wanted to attend community college and begin his first semester taking five classes. His father thought that was too much for him to start with. Adam was furious at this perceived paternal limitation and would never speak to his father again. Sure of himself and what he wanted, Adam wrote his college entrance essay on why pedophilia should be permitted, submitting a 34-page, researched, historically accurate and informed essay on this topic. He also wrote a screenplay about a pedophilic affair between a 10-year-old boy and a 30-year-old man. We recall that Adam's parents divorced when he was 10 years old.

Adam would drop out of community college, often having tantrums and screaming fits before an exam, which would frighten his mother. He would never leave the house except for his trips to the mall, where he played violent video games, sometimes all day without pause. These included *Call of Duty*, a war game, and the game at which he was unsurpassed, *Dance Revolution*, where the player places his legs and arms on arrows on a mat, copying a dancer on TV. As if a game without end, Adam played this for 8–10 hours at a time. What was he working at for 10 hours in front of the dancer on the screen, except to make the mirror work and bear the drive energy in the body of a 19-year-old.

Homebound, presumably for his safety, Adam blogged that he often "felt unsafe at home." He became obsessed with the military and, longing to be a marine, wore military gear for months before the attack. Police found documents in his computer entitled "Babies," in which he wrote about being attacked by babies and trying to defend against them. We note the transitivism of psychosis. At the time of the Sandy Hook shootings, Adam Lanza was 6 feet tall and weighed 112 pounds. The autopsy showed signs of brain damage as a result of malnutrition. For all the devoted maternal care, Adam Lanza was starving.

Listening to Adam

About a year before the shootings, Adam called into an anarchist radio show he had been a fan of, entitled "AnarchyRadio," to speak with the show host, John Zerzan. He related the story of Travis the chimp. Big news in Connecticut where it happened, a domesticated chimp attacked his owner's friend as well as his owner. I cite the transcript of the phone call and give you Adam's words:

> Relevant to your interest, I would like to talk about Travis the Chimp. Travis was a highly domesticated chimpanzee brought up in Stamford, Connecticut. He was raised like a human child starting from the week he was born. The incident occurred when he was 14 – which would be 20 in human years [Adam was 20 at the time of the shootings]. He must have had knowledge of his exceptionality. Overweight, raised in a human world, no different than a mentally handicapped child, he stabbed his owner's friend and then, when his owner stabbed him, he looked at her like "Mom, how could you do that to me?" Chimps shouldn't be in civilization. Travis was profoundly sick, watching baseball, computer pictures, taking Xanax! I thought – why did he want to go for a ride? – I figured it out – He wanted his owner to take him somewhere else. It is wishful to see this as the

> senseless violence of a chimp instead of a human, wishful thinking at best. This is entirely parallel to violence everywhere. He could have been a teenage mall shooter.
>
> (YouTube, 2014)

He adds: "The true murderer was the Xanax Travis was on."

Intelligent and articulate, and psychotic, Adam was well aware of the "swindle" that is "social belonging." His sensitivity to the fact that normalcy is only something "aped" was a way he was able to speak his own suffering to the radio show host. We should add that Peter Lanza had moved to Stamford (the home of Travis the chimp), just an hour from Newtown.

The main blog Adam frequented was entitled: "Shocked beyond belief." The title is important; Adam had no interest in belief, since belief is the way others are bound by words and groups, and the way others are duped by fantasy – precisely what was impossible for Adam.

Adam was a keen cultural critic. "Clothes are slaves to civilization," he blogged. Sometimes he sounds like a Buddhist: "The self is a delusion; life cannot be anything other than suffering." But most of the time, civilization is Adam's culprit. "Marriage is a mutually destructive cultural delusion," he writes. He continues:

> Civilization has not been present for 99% of hominid existence. And the only way it is ever sustained is by indoctrinating each new child for years on end. The "wellness" that you speak of is solely defined by a child's submission to this process and their capacity to propagate civilization themselves . . . New children will end up not well . . . In a short time, children will be brain-washed, pumped full of Xanax and told to conform until they are turned into the oppressors. The children are already dead.

Adam writes: "I hate every facet of language along with the entire concept of aesthetics. I hate culture. . . . I want to live any time and place before language infected humans." Culture would soon become life itself. "I hate how I spend 99% of my time upset about culture when life itself is the problem. Culture just adds insult to injury" (quoted in Langman, 2015b). Founding the problem in life allows Adam a way to target the problem.

It is no surprise that Adam waxed philosophical on the Columbine shootings. "Columbine is a popular topic because it allows for speculation. Such speculation would not have existed if Evan and Dylan survived." Adam knew that – like Evan and Dylan – the only way to "allow for speculation" was to die himself; one cannot not be struck by the fact that his father is introduced by Andrew Solomon in *The New Yorker* article (Solomon, 2014) as "not given to speculation."

Up and Adam: the tsumommy of bullets

In the midst of his shooting spree, the 20-year-old in military dress and mask called out at the top of his lungs, "Look at me!" and then, "Come over here and look at them!" pointing towards the dead children on the floor. Shooting, Adam Lanza, the boy who taped up his bedroom windows with garbage bags, finally wanted to be looked at; he wanted to be seen. His act would surpass that of Dylan and Eric. "Look at me!" he yelled, and "look at them!" Adam found a way to say, "yes" in the mirror. He found a way to "be." In less than 5 minutes, he would fire 156 shots, punctuated dramatically by two shots from the Glock (a gun significantly not made of metal) and the gun he reserved for himself, the last shot to his own head. Like any act, Adam's is overdetermined. Decompleting the Mother, he is trying to invent a self. Shooting, he is finally someone to be looked at, and he made sure the world would see him.

Adam's act made others suffer like he did; others would have to question their beliefs and their "faith" in the system, and the "security" and "safety" of the family-oriented small Connecticut town. To shock others "beyond belief" is a desire to make a trauma. The Parisian analyst Jean-Jacques Moscovitz, following Lacan, has theorized that the psychotic tries to "install a trauma" (Moscovitz, 2005). Trauma is real; belief requires doubt. In some way, we could see the shootings as Adam's solution to the problem of belonging – now others would feel the real hole that Adam suffered. They would be like Adam: without a place to belong, in front of death without the "comfort" of belief in a civilization that holds them.

Obsessed with the "mass" in "mass murder," what I call the "tsumommy" of bullets, is a cataclysmic incarnation of the underside of language, of language as Real, of the impact of the Symbolic, making a hole in the Real. On the one hand, by his act, Adam attested to the fact that "mass murder" was a form of "self-actualization," and on the other hand, he emphasized that there was "no self" to "actualize." These are not mutually exclusive positions. Indeed, we should see mass murder as an attempt to construct an ego and an inscription, and to inscribe the "mass" that traversed him that was only too successful.

Poised against language, life and culture, at the same time, in this very position, he is paradoxically condemned to take culture's most lethal form. The fight against language's killing the thing, he can only really kill the Thing. We could add that Adam might have seen himself paradoxically as sparing the children growing up and becoming separated beings of culture. Here he is also acting out his mother's wish to keep children forever children.

School is a privileged locus of separation as well as a place where knowledge is imparted. School is the venue of symbolic separation as well as real separation from one's parents, a move that was not possible for Adam except in his death. And yet, Adam is right: only in the Real is separation ultimately fully possible. This act of killing, however, has the paradoxical function of making the Mother complete at the same time. Homebound, Adam is finally dead, like his mother. With her and separated from her, dead, finally belonging with the other murdered children at his school.

Finally, Adam made sure no one would touch him and there would be no more noise.

Adam and evil: look to the children!

"Look to the children . . . all of you!" Fritz Lang warns us at the end of his classic 1931 *M*, alerting us throughout the film of our own desire to kill, of our own civilized inheritance – that is, of our position as metaphoric child murderers, having "murdered" the child in us to join "civilization."

Andrew Solomon asked Peter Lanza what they had done about a funeral for Adam. "No one knows that," Peter replied, "And no one ever will" (Solomon, 2014). The secret of Oedipus's burial at Colonus allowed the founding of the city of Athens. Athens is founded on the burial of Oedipus. And the secret lies with Theseus to be transmitted to other civic leaders; a city and transmission is founded over the burial place where Oedipus is laid to rest.

And Adam? "No one knows; and no one ever will." No secret, no city, no future, no transmission, no Oedipus, no Sophocles. And yet, we might wonder if "no one knows," but at the same time, perhaps somewhere we all do. Unlike a secret that can be transmitted, this "knowing" remains a secret both to ourselves and to speech. It does not concern a secret that can be told, but a secret that, in being told, can never be said. This is what Lang's film makes so clear – the kinder murderers are the criminals who bare the very worst of the criminals' hate; indeed, they are the ones whom everyone hates. Peter Lorre as Hans Beckert cries out in that heart-wrenching monologue, "Who knows what it's like to be me!" Lang's film shows that no one knows, and that somewhere, everyone knows. We don't know from Adam and we know from Adam both mean the same thing.

References

Boeckler, N., Seeger, T., Sitzer, P., et al. (eds.). (2013). *School Shootings: International Research, Case Studies, and Concepts for Prevention.* New York, Heidelberg, Dordrecht, London: Springer.

Centers for Disease Control. (2016). *School Violence: Data & Statistics, Understanding School Violence – Fact Sheet.*

Cullen, D. (2010). *Columbine.* New York: Hachette.

FBI (2014). Report cited in Office of the Child Advocate, State of Connecticut: Shooting at the Sandy Hook Elementary School. November 21, 2014.

Freud, S. (1930). *Civilization and Its Discontents. The Standard Edition of the Complete Psychological Works of Sigmund Freud (S.E.)* XXI. London: Hogarth Press. pp. 59–145.

Freud, S. and Einstein, A. (1978) *Why War?* Chicago Institute for Psychoanalysis.

Langman, P. (2010). *Why Kids Kill: Inside the Mind of School Shooters.* NewYork: St. Martin's Press.

——. (2015a). *School Shooters: Understanding High School, College and Adult Perpetrators.* Lanham, MD: Rowman & Littlefield.

——. (2015b). The enigma of Adam Lanza's mind and motivations for murder. *The Journal of Campus Behavioral Intervention, 3*, pp. 1–11.

Lieberman, J. A. (2008). *School Shootings: What Every Parent and Educator Needs to Know to Protect Our Children.* New York: Citadel.

Morel, G. (2008). *La loi de la mere: Essai sur le sinthome sexuel.* Paris: Economica.

Moscovitz, J.-J. (2005). L'écoute diagnostique. Sur les entretiens préliminaires avec un analysant et 'sa psychose. *Psychologie Clinique*, 20: 157–167.

Newman, K. S. (2005). *Rampage: The Social Roots of School Shooting*. New York: Basic Books.

Office of the Child Advocate, State of Connecticut. (2014). *Shooting at the Sandy Hook Elementary School*. November 21, 2014.

Rabin-Havt, A. (2016). Two dangerous weapons: guns and lies. *Lies, Incorporated: The World of Post-Truth Politics*. New York: Anchor Books.

Solomon, A. (2014). The reckoning: the father of the Sandy Hook killer searches for answers. *The New Yorker*, March 17.

Winnicott, D. W. (1946). "Children's hostels in war and peace: a contribution to the symposium on 'Lessons for child psychiatry'." Paper presented at a meeting of the Medical Section of the British Psychological Society, February 27.

——. (1964/1986). This feminism. *Home Is Where We Start From: Essays by a Psychoanalyst*. London: Penguin. pp. 183–193.

YouTube. (2007). "Seung-Hui Cho Full Video Virginia Tech Shooter" (online video clip), April 24.

——. (2014). "Adam Lanza 2011 Call into World Anarchy Radio Travis the Chimp" (online video clip), January 16.

Ziv, S. (2014). *The Register*, November 25.

6

THE TORTURED CHILD

Franz Kaltenbeck

A shocking number of children today are subjected from an early age to the most unspeakable violence: mistreatment, abuse, torture, involuntary and voluntary manslaughter. Assessing the National Institute of Health and Medical Research numbers in 2013, Anne Tuzs estimates that "two children on average . . . die every day from violence inflicted by adults, usually by their parents."[1] They become prey to the perverted, destructive drive of adults. Whereas some children are pampered, adored most often by the blind love and devotion of their parents, even idealized and cosseted, whether adored or abused, children can rapidly lose their human status. Outlawed, they become beings whose bodies and lives are dependent upon their father's, mother's or other relatives' every whim. Nobody henceforth will intervene in their lives and inescapable fates. Uncles, aunts, grandparents do not see the injuries caused by beatings, nor the bruises, open wounds or scars. Father, mother, brother, sister, friends . . . not one of these symbolic names or social links work to protect or care for these children. They cannot even rely on the respect one owes to enemies.

Beyond a certain point, even children's tormentors cannot look at them any more. In an example from my own clinical practice, a mother, having hit, beaten and relentlessly attacked her 5-year-old daughter, could not bear to look at her stricken body, not even having realized that the child had just died from the blows she had inflicted. And for society, beyond the family circle and neighbors, sometimes even for teachers and doctors, these children disappear from the safeguard and safety nets of all social services, become zombies and are avoided by their brothers and sisters.

As in the case of many disasters, child abuse occurs unexpectedly despite an obvious build-up, as nobody sees anything happening. The perpetrators trigger a cycle of violence which they soon lose control of because no child can resist them.

It seems that violence demands still more violence in what is often an endless cycle. Those close to the children look away. The victims are too small, too weak and isolated to be able to perceive the warning signs of what is about to happen to them and thus escape, even if their anxiety has already warned them of a dark threat.

In another clinical example, a mother, guilty of having killed her daughter, would often refer to the tornadoes and their paths of destruction in her country when she talked of her actions when overcome by blind rage.

Until further notice, society remains too passive to prevent the worst from happening. However, the inexorable unfolding of events leading to irreversible damage, repeats itself in a number of similar points from one case to the other and allows us to describe *constants* in the case of children fated to suffering and eventually death. One can thus observe a chain reaction: children are deprived of any love they might have had and become creatures abused in the name of discipline or brutal education; they are more and more estranged, isolated, then imprisoned and finally excluded from the human community, this exclusion allowing the deadliest of acts.

The weaker they get, the more children are hidden, and even if they are seen from time to time, they are no longer perceived as human beings. These children have become shadows or wraiths, vegetating out of sight.

In many ways, the tortured child has been banished to a cruel exile. He is in a prison camp for him alone, a private prison in which he is the only prisoner.

Abuse is similar to a nightmare but without sleep's anaesthetic properties. It may begin with the arrival in a child's life of a stranger, whom he will not realize fast enough bears him ill will. Another child's family life and its fragile equilibrium will be stripped away, and he will learn only to expect to be repeatedly hit.

What is the onset, what are the patterns of abuse which we could identify before it is too late? We must be wary of hasty conclusions, such as expecting that an unwanted child is fated to maltreatment. It is a common explanation given by many, often by the perpetrator, for the abuse inflicted upon their offspring. A lifetime's experience and an open-ended psychoanalysis may prevent us from falling into the trap of such justifications. Since when have the difficulties of desire caused an escalation of violence?

We must, however, seriously consider complaints from the perpetrators of child abuse of their having themselves suffered abuse. They have often been violently beaten during their childhood or as teenagers. When these subjects disclose the trauma to a doctor or therapist, they should be advised to seek counselling when they themselves become fathers or mothers. Another warning sign is when a child is from birth treated as an easily disposable object, according to libidinal investments, to the conflicts of the parents or to the varying fates of the family.

The relationship of adults to their child can be perceived in their own speech. It would be better to realize that their child is, in the best of cases, tolerated but never loved. And when a mother has not even understood that she has never been separated from her child or children, she also incurs the risk of rejecting them completely when they start to bother her.

Abuse can begin in different ways. As a clinician who has spent a good part of my career working within the prison system, I have witnessed a multitude of ways in which abuse can manifest. For little Louis, at the age of 5, it was his 30-year-old mother, whom we'll call Olga, meeting a new partner and this man coming to live with them. She was divorced from the father of Louis and his elder brother Xavier, and had raised her children on her own for 3 years. At the beginning, a 40-year-old unemployed man we'll name Basile had been introduced to Olga by a friend of hers and had become her sons' playmate. All was for the best (in the best of worlds). But this man was an alcoholic and a drug addict, and was to be imprisoned several months for driving without a license. On his return, he had completely changed. Had his imprisonment gone badly? Had he suffered from drug withdrawal in jail? We cannot tell, as much of this man's life is unknown.

The abuse started in December. Louis might have been rude to Basile and then been spanked. These "punishments," which Basile took care to justify to the boy's mother, became more and more violent and frequent. "Louis was not allowed to do anything," said his mother during her first interview in prison, as she tried to make me believe that she had condemned her ferocious partner's behavior. The boy's injuries were soon visible. Basile also knew how to manipulate the older brother against the smaller one. Xavier, who was never hurt by him, admonished Louis, who, at night, even from the depths of his agony, would try to excuse himself and beg for forgiveness.

During a holiday in a seaside hotel, Olga and Xavier left Louis under Basile's watch for a few hours. The boy allegedly insulted a hotel patron in a corridor, but this person was never identified by the hotel receptionist or by anybody else. Did this mysterious client ever exist? Or was he a figment of Basile's imagination, so he could then hit the little boy even harder? Or was it a drug-induced hallucination, which could expunge his atrocious acts? It seems that nobody asked him why.

However, it was a turning point in the unfolding of violence because, from then on, the spanking made way to blows or kicks, and the abuse would be relentless. Basile's violence escalated to acts of barbarism. When the details were disclosed in court, several people, including a member of the jury, fainted.

After the first "educational" phase, as Basile would put it, still trying to justify the abuse he inflicted on Louis, he would beat him continually and deprive him of any kind of the freedom or spontaneity that all children need. Everything was forbidden, anything served as a pretext for insane sanctions, justified in the mind of a drug addict whose drug-induced behavior was so ghastly it seemed to belong to one of the abject characters depicted by David Lynch in *Twin Peaks* or *Blue Velvet*.

However, a tormentor never stops, be it by day or by night. Lacan insisted on the limitlessness of the *sadean* tormentor who wants to persecute his or her victim beyond death. It is Saint Fond's fantasy. But the *sadean* limitlessness is not only a fantasy but also a *passage à l'acte* that is here to stay. Suffering in Nazi concentration camps was relentless; in the prisons of Assad, of Daech, torturing is relentless, too. And closer to us, abused children are left to tormentors whose ambiguity makes them feel guilty and unable to feel hatred towards these criminals who strike in the family circle. Henceforth, the families where crime is embedded are not only the *loci* of the uncanny, but also that of a limitless monstrosity.[2]

Indeed, Basile injured Louis so severely that he could no longer walk but was forced to. And when he fainted, Basile and Olga, his mother, would wake him up with cold showers. The open wounds on his face could not be ignored, either by the couple's friends or family. But Olga had a formidable defense to the rare questions raised by outsiders about her hellish home: she was the woman who knew how to care for children. This was all she could do. This reputation misled and silenced everybody, her family doctor first and foremost; she had taken care of his children, so she could not possibly harm her own

And then she had given her son the wild and fantastical diagnosis of having a "split personality" which apparently caused him to self-inflict injuries and made him fall down the stairs. Everybody believed her lies, her family doctor was totally gullible; he did not even ask the boy to undress in order to examine his injuries but referred him to his brother-in-law, who referred him to a child psychiatrist to prevent the boy from self-harm and mutilating his genitals.

Only one woman came close to saving the child. "Who did this to you?" she asked him when she saw his split lip. Louis, crying, replied: "I did not do it," while looking at his torturer, who held him in his arms. By the boy's glance, she immediately surmised what had happened and decided to contact a child protection agency, but she changed her mind a few hours later because it seemed impossible that her friend Olga could have tolerated such cruelty. And as often in disasters, false hope only worsens the victim's nightmare.

Louis died a month after the enigmatic stay in the seaside hotel, when his life took a horrific turn. All the hellish couple's attempts to revive him failed. Basile has only given one answer to the question as to why he continually attacked little Louis, and his feeble excuse is that drugs made him do it. He might have said to the judges that he deserved a death sentence, but he has not admitted responsibility as a subject. He insists that the torturer and murderer are not part of his true nature but rather the result of the cocktail of drugs he had taken before beating the boy. An investigator has asked: "How could this unemployed man have had access to such great quantities of drugs?"

Refusing to explain such terrible actions is the abdication of this man as a speaking subject. Basile did not present himself as a responsible person but as a helpless puppet driven by a drug-fueled body. The tormentor's cowardice was compounded by the passivity of his partner Olga, the boy's mother. She has been indicted and convicted as an accomplice to the crime. Her inability or lack of will to denounce her partner's crimes and save her son's life were the core of the therapeutic interviews I had with her every week during the three years she was on remand – too brief a time for such a serious matter. As with many convicted criminals, the unconscious had great difficulty in overcoming the ego's censorship and could not weaken the subject's self-justifying speech. For a long time, Olga's dreams enabled her to survive in prison. She was mainly concerned to know whether Xavier, her eldest son, would come and see her. Louis would only appear in nostalgic scenes of family life, without being differentiated as the lost object.

Olga could only mourn the life she had lost; she could not mourn the child she had lost. In her dreams, Louis had the same place that he had in the way she spoke of him to me – an afterthought in her life. She would describe him as a boisterous child whose school accommodated him. But at home, he never wanted to leave his mother's side. He could not bear being sent to his grandparents or to other relatives. It was as if he had never been recognized by them and thus anticipated their betrayal during the final month of his ordeal.

Olga would describe Louis as a strong and serious boy, who did not hesitate in getting into fights, whereas Xavier was more discreet and intellectual with a very good school record despite being placed in foster care while she was imprisoned. Louis seemed to be part of her; she could identify with his shyness, and, after his death, he was erased. She could only remember his alleged passivity when facing torture and abuse. She construed him as an enigma, bearing his suffering in silence.

At the beginning of the interviews, she tried to make me believe that she had stood up against her partner's abuse of Louis. According to her, Louis considered Basile as a surrogate father even if his real father came to visit occasionally.

Olga strenuously denied that Louis had ever screamed when he was "punished" by Basile, even when he was being tortured. A child of his age can indeed not feel pain when he is being beaten, but this tolerance does not last long and is based on the equivocal meaning of a slap, which can be interpreted as being part of a game.

Physical punishment, given by responsible parents, can be accepted by their children. Despite my protesting against her crude denial, Olga maintained the fiction of her tortured son's silence as a miracle, but also as a convenient alibi that protected her own passivity. Olga had, however, told an investigator that Louis did not scream because Basile used to order him to keep quiet.

With regards to her being unable to go to the police or to speak to friends or relatives so that she could get help in removing her son from the deadly hold of Basile, she would give several reasons. She was only rarely allowed to go and see her son in his bedroom. She stated ambiguously: "I belonged to Basile." Her greatest fear was that Basile would break her phone and take revenge upon her eldest son or perhaps her own parents. The people close to her, her neighbors, her doctors and her friends working in Louis's school believed in her obscene inventions about his self-harming and his split personality despite his having been previously considered a happy little boy. The unavailability of people who had seen the injuries on Louis's body and who did not intervene; the fear of being accused and being judged as complicit, and of maybe losing both her children; the guilty gullibility of her community that could only comfort her in her cowardice.

And finally, the real reason: after having spent so many years on her own, she could not give up her passion for Basile, and thus she continued to dream on and on in jail about having had "a good relationship" with Basile and still asking her son, Xavier, for forgiveness, having seen her partner again in her dream.

According to the word associations triggered by this dream, she reached the hypothesis that she had given up on Louis because of her satisfying sexual relations with Basile.

"Love makes us blind," she would say and then immediately add, "I convinced myself that what I saw was not true." This "not true" was "made possible" by simply closing the door when Basile tortured her son, so that her eldest son would not witness the beatings. For a long time before finding this explanation – she was still a free woman – she would say to a friend that she was not going to give up her life as a woman and be a mother to her youngest son. This did not stop her from asking why she had not been able to save her son. But it was her destroyed life rather than her son's death that tormented her. She had indeed sacrificed her son to the sadism of the "dark god" embodied by her partner. And for this man, sexual satisfaction would never be enough; he had to torture a child to death.

It is absolutely wrong to infer from the misunderstood works by Wilhelm Reich that sexual satisfaction of the erotic drive could be used as a foundation to the peaceful lives of human beings.

By my encouraging her to yield to total passivity, our interviews gave way to speech where she could say the most shocking and unexpected statements. Hence, this extraordinary utterance: "I was neutral." The truth that escaped her left us speechless. How could she be neutral? She enlightened me to how she had refused to take a stand for her child against his executioner, whom she believed was above others, the arbitrator, the missing third person in the massacre of her son. At that moment she identified with the representatives of society who remained passive in her small town where the tragedy took place. If they failed to act, why should she? There is in this arrogance of taking the place of the missing Other, a megalomaniac dimension, and this also in regards to another one of her hypotheses, that Basile had destroyed Louis because he was jealous of the little man who had won his mother's favours.

Immediately after Christmas, following the hotel episode, someone else had shown concern for the injuries on little Louis's face. This time it was his own father who had come to their home. He asked his son, "Who hit you?"

Louis, paralyzed by the presence of his mother and her partner, could only reply, "Nobody hit me." His father then offered to take Louis out to buy him a Christmas present. But as her ex-husband was drunk, Olga did not want to let Louis go. What she really wanted was to prevent father and son from speaking to each other. And her ex-husband was too weak to insist.

As to the others who could have freed the child from his torture chamber, why did they not act? A journalist made this very apt comment: during his ordeal, nobody looked at Louis, but during the public trial, an increasing number of people would gather in the courtroom to watch the legal proceedings against Basile and Olga.

The story of little Louis is a tragedy, but the tale we have been told describes a child who was far from being a mute and passive, almost stoical victim, as his mother would have it. Two events during his last days prove that he did, in fact, try to resist. He obviously could not defend himself against his tormentor, but on a cold January day, he tried to escape by running away through a field in front of his mother's house. It was useless. Basile could catch him easily. The cruelty he inflicted, which I choose not to give the details of here, incurred wounds that Louis could not possibly survive. He died two weeks later, on January 25. An even more moving image: one day his mother came upon him in his bedroom. He had climbed onto his toy chest to open the window. And through the window he tried to attract the attention of passers-by so that they could save him. Nobody noticed him. His mother derived some comfort in telling this to me.

Louis was sacrificed by his mother to the dark man who was Basile. Did her blind passion for this man really make her abandon her child to a torturer? Would not the link between a mother and her son prove strong enough to resist such abandonment? Yes, probably. But what if the link was too weak, if it ever held anything? After 3 years of interviews and only during our last one before her transfer to another prison, did Olga describe the following nightmare:

> I was at a 5- or 6-year-old child's christening. At the altar, the priest poured some water on his head. The people around us were dressed normally. But when the priest had stopped pouring the water on the child's head, I turned towards the audience in the church, and I realized that there were only men and women dressed in black, while I had come to a christening!

This nightmare leads her from a christening to a funeral. One can interpret the christening ritual in her dream as the cyphering of an act of torture. The priest would thus represent the torturer. Did not this dream tell her that the gift of a name for her son would mean his death sentence? This woman had been very depressed before Louis's birth. Her husband had been violent with her. He had had legal problems, which resulted in a loss of social status, from which he never recovered. Olga's father had already neglected her or even rejected her as a child, and she only saw her mother as a sick woman, a prey to her husband's brutality. Her mother would alleviate her suffering with alcohol. There had never been a proper link between Olga and her own mother. Her depression at Louis's birth was thus overdetermined. Olga defended herself against this depression by turning her aggressive drive against her son.

The last dream she ever had during our interviews was a memory of having just given birth to Louis.

Three years later, Ingrid, a 23-year-old woman, was incarcerated in the same prison and indicted for the involuntary manslaughter of her 5-year-old daughter Vivienne. The charges were changed to voluntary manslaughter when she was remanded in custody. Rémi, Ingrid's partner and father of her daughter aged 1, was also indicted. Ingrid's eldest daughter, whose father was the same as Vivienne's, lived in the same house. I will not dwell on the sinister staging that the couple made up to hide Vivienne's death and for which Ingrid and Rémi were both indicted.

Ingrid comes from a problematic family. Her father is described as violent, hitting his children in public. He would lock up his seven children and take away telephones and even the windows' handles and bring them to his workplace so that the children could not go out and see their friends in the street. Two of the children were placed in foster homes. He had apparently molested them. Ingrid considers her mother immature, almost mentally deficient. A relationship with a young man named Rudy, who was a year older than her when she was barely out of puberty, allowed her to escape the restricted and constrained life she had led in her parents' house. She became pregnant when she was 16 years old and gave birth to Madeleine. Another pregnancy, when she was 17 years old, ended her school education. She did not want the child but Rudy asked that she keep it. After her birth, Vivienne was at first entrusted to the care of Ingrid's mother and later taken back by Ingrid when she was three months old. The couple and their two daughters, having at first lived in their parents' respective homes, moved into their own flat. Living together was difficult: Rudy would get angry with Ingrid and hit her, and continued to do this until Ingrid left with Madeleine to move in with a man she had met at work, Rémi. She left Vivienne to Rudy, and his grandmother took care of her.

In the meantime, Ingrid raised a family with Rémi – Madeleine and a daughter she had with him. Not really grown-up but having a strong character, she hoped for a life far from the poverty and misery she had known. Having had to forfeit her education meant that her daughters would have to compensate for her own failure and do well in school. She thus created a new life for herself, hoping to raise an ideal family. Hence she started missing Vivienne.

Being on bad terms with Rudy, who was living with another woman, she did not have much hope in getting Vivienne back. But Rudy's grandmother allowed her at times to see her daughter. And yet Ingrid was not satisfied with those visiting rights. She experienced Vivienne's absence as a "great injustice." She did not then turn to the law, and soon gave up on hiring a lawyer. Despairing, she felt that the law would never be on her side.

She then decided to take her daughter away from school, and this was the moment that Vivienne's life changed dramatically into unbearable alienation and then into the horror of physical abuse, resulting in her being killed by being beaten and kicked to death by her mother and her mother's partner.

At first, all seemed well: Ingrid had her three daughters with her. This was her right as a mother. She also took revenge on Rudy and his family for having repelled her when she claimed her visitation rights to see her second daughter. She claimed they had even physically attacked her when she came to their house, and according to her, these attacks deserved revenge. She had, by taking Vivienne away, founded a new family by claiming ownership of all three of her daughters. From then on, she could do whatever she wanted to them. "I never could hurt a child who was not mine." But how would she treat her own children? She was at the head of a closed and soon totalitarian household for Vivienne.

A strange linguistic mistake shows under a crude light her relationship to the law. She confused the words "authority" and "authoritarianism." In order to say that she was strict with Vivienne after taking her away from school, she would say: "authority had started (then)."

There were, however, two drawbacks. It was impossible to enrol Vivienne in her new neighborhood school because she had not been officially removed from her previous school. It was only her father, who was legally responsible in case of any changes because he had enroled her, who could disenroll her. At first, Ingrid did not want to ask him to disenroll their second daughter, and when she finally had made up her mind, he refused to act, arguing that he did not even know where Vivienne lived. An attempt at starting legal proceedings was soon abandoned. Vivienne had disappeared from all social safety nets. The police did not get involved and her school did not inquire after her.

Ingrid, never lacking options, kept well out of sight of the public authorities, and took on the role of the schoolteacher for her second daughter, having pushed her eldest daughter, Madeleine, to the top of her class. Fateful arrogance for Vivienne! She closed up during the exams her mother organized to test her knowledge: Vivienne could no longer even spell her father's name, not even her own surname, nor her first name. Ingrid's world was collapsing. Sometimes she regretted having "taken her daughter back." She regretted it because the child "was a failure." Vivienne had lost all attraction for her mother and her utopian ambitions. The dream of a family where everybody would be successful came to an end. The ghost of failure and regression started to haunt the home.

The lessons she had started to give to her daughter two weeks after taking her away from school became humiliating scenes during which Vivienne closed up totally, her trauma having caused her to lose all the cognitive skills she had proven to have had in school. Vivienne and the deficiencies induced by her mother's brutal methods became the center of Ingrid's life. And at the same time, the girl who was considered backward, a failure, started to lose her place in the family. Her mother would say: "She did not ask to be photographed with the others"; "she was already lost before being killed." After every unanswered question, Vivienne would be punished: she was forced to stand in the corner of the room or on the cellar's staircase and spend hours there, hands on her head. If she ever let her arms down, her mother would slap her, the slaps soon becoming blows. Like many children who lack affection, Vivienne would steal sweets from the cupboards. Her mother would then consider her as sly and identify her all the more to Rudy, her father whom she resembled. Vivienne could no longer sleep and would walk about her room after bedtime, and this would bother Ingrid and Rémi who watched TV in the living room under the children's bedroom. Incensed with rage, Ingrid would take Vivienne out of the bedroom and give her cold showers. Her partner witnessed these scenes and did not calm Ingrid down.

Vivienne might have lost her knowledge but not her contradictory character. When her mother would ask her why she was not sleeping, she used to reply: "Because I do not want to!" She refused to admit to stealing, and Ingrid, overcome with rage, would then start beating her daughter and injure her. The only effect Vivienne's promises not to steal from the cupboards and refusing to sleep had on her mother, was a worsening of her mother's temper. Ingrid demanding that her daughter go to sleep is rather curious considering she had reduced her to becoming her very own *punching-ball.* Any vital reaction from this child who was trying to defend herself against death would further increase the fury of Ingrid's destructive drive. The mother would say: "I built myself on anger, on hate"; "the more I punished her, the more I took it out on her." And yet she had herself survived her own father's abuse. Men and women who become the instruments of this kind of death drive do not give any leeway to those who want to live; they crush them.

This is how the last punishment became torture and eventually death for the little girl. Unable to sleep, she had yet again walked to and fro in the bedroom she shared with her sister, Madeleine, who was already asleep. Her mother rushed to take her out of the bedroom and started hitting and kicking her in the bathroom. She put her under the cold shower and hit her repeatedly with the shower head. Vivienne would beg again and again for her mother to stop beating her. The little girl would promise to go to sleep. Her mother would then reply to her: "I know that this is not true!" Vivienne would thus also "die from truth" (Nietzsche, *Beyond Good and Evil* § 4), because of her mother's "madness for truth."

After desperately begging and begging – didn't her mother know that she was lying? – Rémi would hold her tight so that Ingrid could hit her harder and harder. And then the couple left her under the cold shower and continued watching a stupid movie on television. Having heard some kind of noise or thud, Rémi went back to the bathroom. Vivienne had collapsed and was lying in the shower. All attempts to resuscitate her – with more cold showers, with cardiac massage and mouth-to-mouth resuscitation – would fail; there was no longer any pulse.

Ingrid could not look at her dead daughter. She had not looked at her when she was beating her. Vivienne's eyes and gaze were unbearable. In a rare moment of lucidity, Ingrid said: "I never understood Vivienne." Only in a single dream that she had at the beginning of her imprisonment, did she see herself hitting her daughter.

For several weeks, Vivienne was confined, practically locked away. She had been starved and had lost a lot of weight and could therefore not be seen. Before she was killed, she was no longer part of her family or part of the human community. Rémi carried her naked, wounded body into the cellar without covering her with a shroud. Vivienne's corpse would lie there during a whole weekend because Ingrid's third daughter was to be christened the next day. Hadn't she invited all her family, as well as Rémi's family?

The mistreated, tortured child is also abandoned to her solitude so that the parents can live their so-called "normal life" enjoyment and illusions. At the same time, she is surrounded by people who are ashamed of her physical appearance –

by the brothers and sisters, or by indifferent, hostile relatives. Even if Vivienne had not died, she would never have been in a fit state to go to the party. Her face and body would have immediately betrayed her mother's and mother's partner's crimes, and Rémi did nothing to prevent Ingrid from relentlessly hurting her own daughter. In order to get rid of the body, Rémi buried her in a forest. After being arrested and having confessed to the crime, he had great difficulty in taking the police back to the burial site.

Ingrid and Rémi invented a story to explain Vivienne's disappearance. At some point, Ingrid declared having lost Vivienne in the shopping area of her town, never finding her again. The police had to check two hypotheses: first, that of a family crime; second, that of a kidnapping. The couple was soon suspected, all the more as Ingrid was unable to pretend to be stricken by her daughter's disappearance. The investigators, however, had no proof of guilt, and they would take 6 months to lawfully indict the criminal couple. Rémi, rather too optimistically, had thought that "without a body, they have nothing against us."

Ingrid's inability to mourn her daughter has struck more than one of the people who have taken interest in her case. But this coldness is not so easy to interpret. She did indeed have great difficulties in describing her second daughter in terms of saying what she had been like. Murderers can experience delayed mourning. It is also true to say that Ingrid regretted more than anything else not achieving the kind of life that she had hoped for herself and her family.

She would say after two years in jail: "Yes, it is true that we made a stupid mistake." And ambiguously, she would also say that she was unable to express regret and remorse.

We shall not judge her according to her feelings. But the only regret she had during her preventive detention was the break-up of her couple: "Before we were one. We were bound together by the shared secret."[3]

The French national education system does not have any plan of action in cases of suspicious absences of a child from his school. Several relatives who had been invited to the christening did not even know that Vivienne existed. Ingrid's real family was fragile, defective and the children had not been nurtured by their parents' love. This could explain why Ingrid yearned for an ideal family, which she would then enforce. She did not attempt to fulfill a personal ideal, be it professional or intellectual, but she could only strive for an ideal based on a model completely opposite to her own family in which she had grown up with great difficulty. And yet she had remained identified to her authoritarian and violent father who would do all to crush any of his children's attempts to free themselves from their prison-like home. What she considered as her daughter Vivienne's deviant behavior was only an excuse to impose in her home a mixture of totalitarian terror for the child who would not fit in and an appallingly vulgar hedonistic regimen for the rest of the family.

In the space of 3 years, two couples have battered to death a boy and a girl who were both 5 years old. Basile and Ingrid, the two main culprits, are in fact not comparable. Olga and Rémi, however, their respective accomplices, share the same traits: neither reacted in order to stop their partners' sadistic unleashing of violence or to warn a public authority or ask for help. They could have done so. One may wonder if they really wanted to save the children in their care. Obviously, they were not implicated in these crimes for the same reasons as the ones who actually committed them. However, Rémi has also been accused of hitting Vivienne and having held her as Ingrid was beating her.

Basile acted under the influence of drugs. Was it only because of drugs that he tortured a child to death? Who could possibly answer this question? Olga has, however, articulated during our interviews what prevented her from stopping the crime and torture. It was due, less to her fear of her partner, than to her blinding passion for him, which had filled up a great emptiness inside her. She had been raised by a sick and alcoholic mother and rejected by her father, and she had imagined choosing a career as a nanny, and later as an educational helper. The unhappy marriage, during which she bore two children, reminded her of her childhood traumas. Basile came into her life and her son Louis's life, as a providential man. He could hypnotize her and make her obey him.

Ingrid, having grown up under the yoke of a father with paranoid traits, did not find any solace in her mother who was mentally deficient. Very determined but having also identified with a violent father, she wanted to escape her dysfunctional family by having a relationship at too young an age with Rudy. Her second pregnancy at the age of 17 and giving birth to Vivienne was inconvenient. She did not get on with Rudy who started hitting her and she left school. All these ingredients culminated in her criminal acts: reproaching Vivienne for having wasted her youth; revenge against Rudy with whom she had left Vivienne and who resented her demands to see her daughter. A strong character, she tried to make up for all of this after having met Rémi. She had a third daughter with him and decided to establish once and for all a new life. And too bad if she had failed in her own life; her daughters – all three of her daughters – would embody the ideal family, which would *in fine* become a totalitarian state. The family had to be whole. She had to get Vivienne back, even if this meant taking her away from school. But Vivienne, a strong character too, did not comply, and, feeling like a stranger in her mother's home, she stood up against her, doing whatever she wanted. The impossibility of enrolling her into a new school was a death sentence for the child for whom the other of the law would be abolished until the – near – end of her life.

No social welfare or safety nets for Vivienne, the distracted neighbors had forgotten about her; her own father vaguely searched for her; the school in which she had been a good pupil forgot about her. Ingrid suddenly took on the role of a private and nasty teacher, and lost her temper repeatedly because Vivienne could no longer remember anything, not even how to spell her own name, when confronted with her mother's hatred. This forgetting of what she knew reminded Ingrid of the evil caused by her own renunciation of knowledge, which happened when she was pregnant with Vivienne. One can surmise the devastating effects of the trauma by how quickly the little girl lost all knowledge acquired in school.

And yet, her teachers had described her as an average pupil. Ingrid relentlessly attacked her daughter who had lost all phallic appeal and could never fit into the ideal family that Ingrid had wanted to create.

Having become a *waste product*, Vivienne however fought back against her mother to save herself. Showing resistance to death only provoked in Ingrid the cataclysm, which the Freudians have named *destrudo*, the destructive drive. However much she begged or pleaded, this failed to stop Ingrid's hatred and anger. And yet the mother could not look into her own daughter's dead eyes.

We have tried to demonstrate that these two child murders occurred rather like disasters do – that no one had expected them to happen. In a nightmare, Ingrid has in fact compared the worst of her acts to a tornado. But it would be wrong to say that these disasters did not have warning signs or could have possibly alerted the social services.

The automatic, loveless removal of a child from one family to another bodes no good for the child when the family is just a patchwork of people, organized for utilitarian reasons rather than by affection and love. The repetition of abuse between generations makes its recurrence all the more probable. A severe state of depression in the mother before the birth of her child can become an aggressive drive against this very child, as well as the failure of separation. That drug addiction and alcoholism facilitating the collapse of all of a man's defences against his limitless destructive drive, could be what made Basile become little Louis's persecutor and torturer. Yet this is not a sufficient explanation for what happened.

One is left with the silence of the accomplices and the indifference of the others. This is similar to the great collective crimes committed, for example, by the Nazi state. If indeed it is true that under a totalitarian regime it is impossible to express one's convictions if one is not ready to die, the fact remains that many French people saved Jews during the war, whereas very few Germans or Austrians did the same. In a democracy, one risks little by trying to help a threatened child. And yet these children are so often left alone to face their persecutors. Those close to the victims do not react, which implies complicity. What is most striking in these cases of lack of reaction is perhaps denial. One does not want to look at what is in plain sight; one hears screams without taking them seriously; one is witness to extreme violence and one considers this as just an ordinary occurrence. These powerful mechanisms may paralyze the ability to act, but they in no way excuse cowardice, especially from the professionals – teachers, educators, doctors – who are entrusted with the welfare of children.

We have been able to delineate the different stages of abuse, which can occur without anybody seeing anything. The entrance into the child's life of a man or a woman, partner to their father or mother. Utilitarian displacement of the child into the life of a father or mother he or she does not know well. The child considered as the cause of disturbance in the family. The child becomes a scapegoat. The parent believes in correcting him or her. The child is prey to worsening punishment. The adult who usurps authority starts to enjoy ordering the "punishment." His or her sadism claims only more violence. In the meanwhile, the child is out of the reach of the law, a "vagrant" according to Michel Foucault's lesson of January 17, 1973, in *The Punitive Society* (Collège de France conferences 1972–1973). A slave to his family, the child disappears from the world in which he lived (school, neighbors, friends) and becomes invisible to those who continue to encounter him. The master signifiers "family," "parents," "father," "mother," "brother" . . . do not protect the child but rather protect the persecutors. Are they not the names of sanctuaries, which are hidden and safe from any form of inquiry? The child is reduced to this *waste product* to be gotten rid of in the end. The family has not become the place of this imaginary formation that Freud named the uncanny, but the place of monstrosity where nightmares become real.

Notes

1. Gaëlle Dupont, "Maltreated children: two deaths a day," in *Le Monde*, Saturday, June 15, 2013, p. 11.
2. Or rather, it is a pleonasm. According to Jean-Claude Milner, the social unlimited (social politics) *is* monstrous.
3. Secret of the criminal act. "It was as if something was binding us together." Let us suppose they could have kept the secret. In this case, they would indeed be forced to stay together, each being able to denounce himself or herself or to denounce the other if he or she would not have been able to bear the separation. But after Vivienne's death, Olga also wanted to flee on her own to escape the dyad she now had formed with Rémi, "in which each of them was consumed by their crime."

7

CLICK AND DESTROY

The clinic of video games[1]

Vincent Le Corre

For a psychoanalyst to talk about video games today is not easy. First, because of the current opinion which regularly blames gaming for the most spectacular kinds of violence. Without entering into the discussion – albeit highly relevant – of the artistic merit of video games, the gaming industry itself has launched into an active process of cultural legitimization.[2] However, this mainstreaming is not without its ambiguities: it transforms gaming from a quasi-underground activity of the select few – the geeks – into a socially exponential practice and, as a result, a public enemy number one, thus giving it a truly perilous visibility.

This double process of legitimization and gaining market share has been accompanied by the growing community of gamers, who are also trying to be heard against the discourse that tends to label video games as simply a risk for youth. This collective sensitivity vis-à-vis video games tends to complicate our efforts: some might accuse us of proselytizing, when we speak about the positive characteristics or aspects of gaming, especially as a tool of mediation or psychotherapy, while others will not appreciate us criticizing their less laudable features. The second reason, more fundamental but often ignored, is that it is difficult to clearly define the outlines of our object of study, as Mathieu Triclot's book *Philosophie des jeux video* (*The Philosophy of Video Games*) demonstrates in a highly interesting way (Triclot, 2011, pp. 13–14).[3]

First, we should thus say that the question of video games has today become a complex social fact, which requires a critical and detailed sociological approach, rather than simply a psychological or psychoanalytic examination. We therefore need to combine the "psy" discourse with other discourses in order to study the topic seriously and associate, for example, a clinical analysis with an analysis of the game's contents or the ideologies underpinning them. We also must learn to distinguish between the different practices of video games. Playing on a computer, a living-room console, on one's phone or a mobile console, at school, at home or at a gaming arcade, focusing on games that are played alone and have highly elaborate scenarios, or playing online – these do not refer to the same reality and, as a result, to the same clinic of video games.

The subject of video games has entered the clinical field gradually, first through psychopathology – namely, driven by the media discourse transmitting a kind of moral panic. Gaming is generally associated with several perceived risks: the confusion between reality and fiction; with leading fragile individuals to behaviors that remove them from social life; with the risks of addiction and finally with a link to violent conduct.[4] There is no scientific consensus as to the possible "addiction to video games." Since 2012, the French Medical Council has thus instead used the term "excessive practices."

Based on an account of an encounter with a young patient, I would like to suggest several possible directions of how we may think about the clinical facets of this cultural phenomenon. As we shall see, French psychoanalysts have been interested in video games mainly in connection with the questions of narcissism[5] and the image (Tisseron, 2006). This is the first aspect I will therefore explore. Subsequently, I will look at some aspects of the discourse about the violence of video games. Finally, I will suggest other possible directions, which will emphasize the symbolic dimension and the relationship to the digital machine.

Video games, narcissism and adolescence

Video games are part of the great movement of the history of technology, in which humans continue to try to substitute their natural environment with an environment made purely of representations, where they can feel more in control and thus safer. This movement began as a speculative thought (the omnipotence of the Western mind is sometimes palpable in its philosophy and theoretical systems) and then was gradually realized via technological frameworks. It seems to me that this touches on the question of narcissism and the function of the ideal.

In his article "Reconstruction narcissique du moi adolescent" ("The narcissistic reconstruction of the adolescent ego"), the psychoanalyst Serge Lesourd writes that "the ego, as an object of love, is at the heart of the identity reconstruction in adolescence. At the foundation of narcissism and self-esteem, this ego-object is one of the crucial objects of adolescence" (Lesourd, 2004, p. 28). Faced with the definitive disappearance of the infantile love-object in puberty, the subject needs to try to find it again. In his article, Lesourd makes a distinction between the object of reality, the psychic object of the drive, and another form of psychic object, the ego-object, which is key to the psychoanalytic work with adolescents. Ultimately, it is by creating new objects in reality, but also by manipulating and appropriating real cultural objects, that the re-creation of the ego-object discussed by Lesourd can occur.

Following the same perspective and in order to subvert the paucity of the commonly used binary between the real and the virtual, the psychiatrist and psychoanalyst Serge Tisseron confronts the different meanings of the term "virtual" with the different dimensions of the processes of adolescence (Tisseron et al., 2006, pp. 93–97):

- *The virtual as the future and a contrast with the present*: like in the biological metaphor of the grain that will grow into a tree, the adolescent is an adult in the making. Tisseron therefore identifies a temporal reference framework.
- *The virtual as potentiality, as already there but not yet actualized*: this time, we can take the example of the subject's identifications, which manifest in certain circumstances. This perspective tells us that, faced with, for example, anxiety-provoking situations, the adolescent can either rely on secondary identifications in the same way they would have been used in childhood, or instead he can start using other identifications that will lead him to act as an adult. This framework of reference tends to be spatial, topical, as we could say. An example from the sphere of video games would be the way in which adolescents play with the avatars they construct.[6]
- *Finally, the opposition between the virtual and the corporeal.* Adolescence is indeed a moment in which the question of the body is raised with great urgency on all three planes: in the symbolic, the imaginary and the real. The question of the relationships between the body and the mind is often fantasmatically transformed, using the cultural referents the adolescent is able to mobilize in the culture he belongs to. This also brings up the question of narcissism. Puberty leads to real bodily changes and these in turn result in a change of the body's symbolic status. The body is no longer a child's body, and the adolescent perceives this transformation in the way he is seen by adults. His body is now equal to theirs. Moreover – and this is often the source of family conflicts – it is now possible to implement fantasies both incestuous and parricidal. All this creates serious problems for the adolescent's relationships to his primary objects. These bodily changes lead to what Jean-Jacques Rassial calls "an après-coup of the mirror stage" (Rassial, 1996, pp. 45–54). The recognition of one's own image in the mirror is not easy. Faced with all this, the virtual space and the relationship to the body it offers – namely, the possibility of substituting, in order to play, the "virtual signifier" (the game character or avatar[7]) for one's real body that has become so bothersome, can constitute a way of "taking back control" over what the adolescent may perceive as, precisely, out of his control, thus temporality "bracketing" certain fears of puberty.

"Rewriting the history of video games"

The young man I worked with was a regular visitor at a youth center and could be described as "dependent on video games." Already undergoing psychotherapy, he had agreed with his therapist that he would come to see me for a weekly mediation session "about computers." Quickly, he decided to present to me a project that had already been occupying him for some time, "rewriting[8] the history of video games."

He would then come to each session with several games, which he brought on a USB stick, and was eager to show to me. In our meetings, the computer and the game he would install on it served as a third object and the focus of our gaze. This would result in a situation of shared attentiveness, similar to what we could observe between a young child and an adult (Virole, 2011). The adolescent was playing in my presence and used the game to speak to me. As for myself, I would sometime lose my ability to think, when absorbed by the progress of the game. I assume that this was the same state that he was looking for himself, when he would sometimes play alone at home, for hours on end.

To return to Tisseron's opposition between the virtual and the corporeal, the young man's body was massive, but he was very clumsy. His awkward movements and a constant effort to hide himself betrayed a great fragility. During the game, the picture would change completely: his clumsiness disappeared, and he showed an extraordinary dexterity in manipulating the keyboard or the joystick. When he started playing, there was an effect of offloading, of relief. His heavy body was transformed into the bobbing character on the screen, moving at an extreme speed like the legendary Sonic hedgehog of Sega games, who was one of his favourite characters.

With regards to this, we have to keep in mind that the gaming experience is indeed a bodily experience. Regardless of the interface in question, the player must first subject his body to the requirements of the machine. When using a joystick or a keyboard, we are, of course, involving the hands; when using motion sensors, we use other parts of the body. But the game experience, perhaps more intensely when the interface makes less demand on our body, displaces the way in which we subjectivize our own body. The psychoanalyst Benoit Virole explains this by the fact that "movement intention is projected into the virtual act" (2011, p. 5). He suggests that we frequently observe the calming effect that gaming has on children whose usual hyperactivity conceals an underlying depression.

This young man was especially fond of arcade games, as he had a hard time tolerating the slowness of adventure games, which require thought and careful consideration of the game situations. The games he was playing were therefore games which instead required the construction of automatic behaviors and reflexes in order to progress and continue controlling the hero in an environment that generates an increasingly more frenetic flurry of activities, so that the player must ultimately always lose against the machine.[9]

For this young man, continuing to fight against this infernal machine that was making him lose was a definite pleasure. Lose – but lose in style! His gaming style – i.e., the way he handled his character and the latter's aesthetics – were indeed very important to his enjoyment of the game. The hero, who he thought represented him, was exactly the opposite of his own physique; it was easy to guess that the image he loved to manipulate through the keyboard and which represented him on screen was an idealization of the bodily ego[10] – i.e., the ideal ego. We find here the idea suggested by the psychoanalyst Michael Stora, of the "hand as the metaphor of the ego" (Stora, 2003, p. 21), but also the theorization of the psychoanalyst Frederic Tordo, who coined the notion of "virtual self-empathy."[11] The question of narcissism is therefore key to the problematic of video games.

Violence, did you say violence?[12]

As I said in the introduction, the effects of gaming on subjects and their violent behavior are just as controversial as the risk of addiction supposedly inherent to this activity. We can thus find authors who claim that video games lead our children to kill, to paraphrase the title of a book by Dave Grossman (Grossman and Degaetano, 2014) and others that highlight the cathartic functions of this medium.

First, let us leave this normative vision aside and instead adopt the perspective of Benoit Virole, who on one hand decries the hypocrisy of our societies, which are outraged by the violence in the virtual worlds while themselves constantly promoting aggressive or even predatory economic behavior, especially in the sphere of work; on the other hand, he reminds us that the loss of all initiation rituals drives our young people to look for situations that are, precisely, a symbolic staging of the combat as a field in which to appropriate one's own power. The popular war games such as *Counter Strike* are a good example of this, given the "team work, cooperation and the collective integration of individual qualities" (Virole, 2011, p. 71) they require.

Judging from the latest research carried out by epidemiologists or social psychologists on the links between violent gaming and violent acts perpetrated by gamers, we might find ourselves in a tight spot. There does seem to be a link between the fact of playing a violent video game and several different consequences, such as emotional desensitization (a banalization and a reduction in the sensitivity towards victims), a loss of inhibition regarding violent behavior or the development of a pessimistic worldview.[13] However, the connection between these same video games and the fact of perpetrating criminal acts cannot be established and some authors even associate video games with a decline in criminality (Fournis et al., 2015, p. 173; Cunningham et al., 2011; Ward, 2010).

The point is not to deny that violent games do have effects on their players, even if the question of how to measure these effects remains suspended. Yet another question, perhaps more important, is to ask *why* certain individuals might be attracted to video games in the first place.

I will not attempt, as Lacan already did in his article "Aggressiveness in psychoanalysis" (Lacan, 2005), to try to review the results of the experiments in social psychology in the light of psychoanalytic theory. But following in Lacan's footsteps, I would simply like to emphasize the link between narcissism (and thus the practice of video games) and certain violent acts.

In his article, Lacan indeed articulates the question of narcissism to his arguments about aggressiveness, suggesting that we must "accommodate our thinking if we are to understand the nature of aggressiveness in man and its relation to the formalism of his ego and objects" (Lacan, 2005, p. 92). He argues that "the notion of aggressiveness as a tension correlated with narcissistic structure in the subject's becoming allows us to encompass in a very simply formulated function all sorts of accidents and atypicalities in that becoming" (p. 95). His view is then that prior to the establishment of the Oedipus complex as a "identificatory reshaping of the subject" (ibid.), there exists a first alienating identification, described in his Mirror Stage, which in a sense provides energy for the secondary identification with the rival bound to occur in the Oedipus complex. This secondary identification with the father hence leads to the creation of an agency that Lacan later describes as symbolic, the ego-ideal. In the absence of "the 'pacifying' function of the ego-ideal" (ibid.), the subject remains with this first imago, the "visual Gestalt of his own body" (ibid., p. 90), which he projects on to others, but which can very quickly become persecutory in return.

In the case of school shootings committed by adolescents (in addition to there being statistically more gamers than non-gamers), it is therefore not surprising that the practice of gaming (precisely when it is excessive), which so strongly engages a subject's narcissism, can be found among the perpetrator's activities prior to the crime. Based on Lacan's argument, this crime itself could be interpreted as a form of a violent reaction, linked by him to the "original organization of ego and object forms" (ibid., p. 90) that we find in the psychoses.

Does gaming push the subject to imitate or reproduce the act of killing? Or is it an attempt at producing a supplementation (*suppléance*) on the part of psychotic subjects, providing them with a dyadic relation, to use Serge Tisseron's expression? Drawing on object-relations theory, Tisseron has suggested that the player and the machine indeed create a "digital dyad" (2006, pp. 111–116; Tisseron, 2009). The subject is trying to reproduce, with the machine, a relationship as alienating as the one he had with his primary object, but at the same time also searching for a connection that would be more satisfying and pacifying.

Rather than looking for the cause of these types of violent acts in video games, we should perhaps instead be trying to find out what the young people make of these games and images, what they do with them, and if they have people in their lives with whom they can speak about what they experience and feel. Children or adolescents who are struggling with difficult situations, who have no one to talk to about what they are going through, quickly feel betrayed by adults, and can try to look for other places of refuge and seek other values and reference points – for example, in peer groups. Faced with the violence of their experience, they might have to silence their pain and try to become desensitized to it, particularly through images, and thus try to keep this pain under control.

In her article *Images fictives violentes et thérapies d'enfants: obstacle ou support pour la symbolisation* (Brun, 2008), the psychoanalyst Anne Brun examines the role played by violent fictional images, especially from video games, on the basis of their function in child psychotherapy. For her, working on the impact of these violent images means to question first of all, what it is that these children are looking for in these images, and what is the reason for their quasi-compulsive consumption. For some, they are "a way of linking their traumatic experiences, of trying to externalize them in the perceptive register in order to figure and somewhat diffuse their traumatic charge" (p. 78). She connects the children's need for these images to the family dynamic, especially the parental symptom, and "what cannot be represented in the family" (p. 81). As for the reasons for resorting to these violent images, Brun suggests several hypotheses. In some cases, the child is protecting himself from an intrusion of reality, especially from any intervention coming from the therapist, because he is caught up in "the parents' impossible mourning for an imaginary child" and has been tasked with supplementing the parent(s)' mourning or depression. In other cases, "the child would clutch onto violent fictional scenarios in order to block out the possible arrival of an unthinkable and non-representable experience" (p. 77). These images are therefore asked to "plug a representational hole" but also and simultaneously to try to figure these same primordial anxieties, which Winnicott describes in his *Fear of Breakdown* (Winnicott, 1974).

On the topic of adolescents left without a proper interlocutor, David Michôd's 2011 film *Animal Kingdom* paints a striking portrait of a family ruled by a perverse law, with a young man struggling after the loss of his mother, who finds no one he can trust enough to speak about his pain. In another register, this also seems to have been the case for Adam Lanza, who found it impossible to find anyone with whom he could share his distress. His crime also seems to have been preceded by a period of excessive gaming (Steinkoler, 2016). I will come back to this idea of excessive playing later.

This search for an interlocutor, for someone to talk to and possibly contain and metabolize, with the help of another trustworthy person, experience that has so far remained unthinkable, also chimes with Lacan's remark about the pacifying dimension of the ego-ideal. I will illustrate this via a clinical case.

The use and abuse of the digital object

The imaginary dimension of video games should not obscure the fact that these objects are cybernetic frameworks, which emerged at a certain moment in the history of computing and from specific environments and ecosystems. Within this history, it was only after J. C. Licklider formulated his notion of a man–computer symbiosis (Robert, 2011),[14] later concretized by hackers, that individuals could form a close relationship with the digital machine and video games were born. In other words, these games have an intimate and specific connection to the computer machine that we are familiar with today and that gives us access to a symbolic computational space, including a space for play[15] – to "the computational world," to use the title of a book by the philosopher Jean-Michel Salanskis (2011).

In Triclot's analysis, the minimal component of the video game is this possibility to displace the symbolic space of the rules of the game to a virtual space fully managed by a machine, in order to play with the strange form of "digital matter," ontologically a form of mathematical writing ("discrete, finite and dynamic," as Salanskis puts it). Video games can therefore be seen as a "digital matter" that is to be invested, interacted with, that is produced by the symbolic machine (the computer or the console) and can be grasped as a kind of partner. This digital matter is the locus of an encounter with pliable objects[16] that we can act upon, that we can co-construct, transform and shape thanks to this partner. In return, the possibility of "manipulating" this digital matter can shape certain psychic processes.

Yet that is not all. The computer machine can be used and, above all, abused, because it responds so unfailingly to our requests.[17] Programming in a language brings us into a direct relation with the nature of this matter, while a video game gives us an imaginary perspective on this matter, while preserving some of its key aspects, mainly the possibility to "save" one's position, which means, for example, that a game sequence can be played again and again (Triclot, 2011, pp. 19–23). A certain pleasure can also be drawn from the possibility of experimenting with a potentially creative repetition,[18] using this automatic response provided by the digital matter, understood as the site and the object produced by the machine as the symbolic partner. In the therapeutic relationship, the digital object as an object of mediation can therefore bring to the surface or highlight certain aspects of the psychic reality, which are linked to, on one hand, the characteristics of this digital matter and, on the other hand, the type of relationship that a subject can have with these symbolic machines.

Interpassivity and the symbolic order

Let's now look at this intimate relationship between a subject and a machine during the play experience of the video game. The philosopher Slavoj Žižek coined the notion of *interpassivity* to critique modern-day political activism, which, he argues, consists in a frantic activity intended to ensure that, paradoxically, nothing changes.[19] He uses this notion as an opposing concept to interactivity, which is, of course, at the heart of the question of video games.

During his first seminars, Lacan continued to develop his distinction between the specular ego and the subject, which he sees as linked to the symbolic and which is later elaborated using his theory of the signifier. Lacan's theory presents us with a "de-centred subject": what is most intimate to us is what is indeed constantly escaping us. In the 1960s (once the "big Other" was decompleted), Lacan produced an original definition of the subject – namely, that "a signifier represents the subject for another signifier." Žižek's notion of interpassivity is founded on this notion of the subject whose inner, intimate sphere is ultimately displaced outwards by the signifier's intervention, in other words, through the Other represented as the place where our speech takes on meaning, "the treasure trove of signifiers," but also the "locus of the code."[20] We have seen that the video game is nothing but a computer program encoded in a particular language.

Žižek suggests that we think of the possibility of representing ourselves in a cybernetic space via a character or an avatar using what he calls the "primordial substitution," which is none other than the mechanics of the symbolic theorized by Lacan – i.e., the substitution of a signifier for the subject summarized in his famous formula.[21] "This substitution is the constitutive gesture of the symbolic order: a signifier is precisely something that is substituted for the ego, that acts in our place" (Žížek, 2003, p. 105).[22]

Based on this primordial substitution, Žížek conceives of his notion of the *subject-supposed-to-believe* – in other words, the possibility for a subject to delegate his belief; the Other can believe in the subject's place, such as when parents can continue to believe in Santa Claus through their children. It can also help us understand the "old riddle of the transposed/displaced emotions of professional mourners" (p. 104) or the phenomenon of "canned laughter" on television, the fact that we can "suffer and pay for a sin *via* the Other" and more generally can transfer our emotions, dreams and anxieties to the Other. In trying to participate in the symbolic order, the signifier itself "in its material exteriority" therefore acts in the subject's place,[23] like the character replacing the player in the space of the video game.

With Gregoire Latry (Le Corre and Latry, 2013), we have previously suggested that we consider three levels of symbolization of the player's actions in the framework of the video game, based on the hypothesis that the representations taken from the video game and the video game space could be used to give new form to actions and transform them in the therapeutic group using the video game. On the first level, actions directly represented by the framework of the video game[24] would then be immediately symbolized in the game space.[25] This can be related to Žížek's idea that the character, the avatar or any other virtual object supplied by the game (such as the ball in the 1980s classic *Marble Madness*) as a signifier that substitutes itself for the player's actions, inscribes them on this "other scene," the symbolic space of the game.

To come back to the young man I was working with, beyond the interpretation that would simply see the game character as the representation of his ideal ego, we could now argue that his project of "rewriting the history of video games" was also an urgent effort to inscribe his actions in the symbolic space managed by the machine, by using and abusing the possibility of representing himself in these gaming worlds.

The place of the "little others" in the symbolic–video–play–space

The young man often spoke about his passion for video games as something that had literally saved his life. "Without video games, I'd have already been found dead, I'd have blown out my brains somewhere." I saw this relationship to the game, which he presented as vital, as a kind of escape he had created in the midst of complicated family dynamics, faced with the impasses presented at the time by the confrontation with his peers, but also with his own body and his specular image. Despite strong inhibitions and anxiety, he continued trying to make contact with certain others he saw as benign – for example, through online gaming. He told me that he had started developing "mods"[26] for the game *Doom* and offer them to the community of players, although he detested the fact that he was unable to know whether his creations were popular, whether the other members appreciated them or not.

He would often complain of players who did not respect certain rules during online game sessions. In his view, too many players would use specific techniques to win at all costs; in other words, they exploited what could be seen as faults in the game's programming code. In his experience of the game, "fair play" was a particularly important element. "If you don't take your adversary into account, you destroy the game experience!" he would say. He was so sensitive to this dimension of playing with the other that he began to draft a "code of conduct" for one of the online games.

"The machine [usually] takes care that the rules are respected and the necessary calculations are made; it ensures a form of objectivity or neutrality of the playing field" (Triclot, 2011, p. 39). But the logic of the machine, the "locus of the code," to use Lacan's expression, were not sufficiently neutral or objective for this young man, who said he wanted to guarantee a game space where everyone could have fun fighting one another. In this way, he was trying to restore the space of play normally taken care of by the machine's computational processes, with supplementary rules that everyone should obey and which to his mind would give everyone a fair chance at winning.

The locus of the code and the symbolic law

For this adolescent, video games, their symbolic worlds, but also their history represented a bridge towards culture more generally. Yet they were above all part of his search for the existence of an Other who would guarantee a place for others – an Other he needed yet whose presence, gaze, but also disappearance he feared. The "code of conduct" suggested that he was trying to defend himself against his own destructiveness – i.e., against the aggressiveness that could fantasmatically destroy these others. The "pacifying function of the ego-ideal" I evoked earlier is thus here connected to his effort of trying to overcome the narcissistic impasse.

Thus, we could interpret this "code of conduct" as his attempt to pacify the video game space, considered as a purely symbolic space in which each subject is represented by a "virtual signifier" for another "virtual signifier" – the video–play–symbolic space. This space is pacified by becoming regulated, so that everyone finds their place guaranteed by the symbolic law ensured by the code (the game code) and complemented by a set of rules. This was, of course, something that this young man was unable to find in his daily life, where the mediation of the symbolic law guaranteed by a sufficiently consistent Other seemed to be lacking, plunging him into anxiety.

For the player, the video–play–symbolic space [*l'espace video–ludo–symbolique*] can, in fact, bring the Other into existence, as the philosopher Maxime Coulombe noticed when he tried to immerse himself in the *World of Warcraft* community.[27] While the young man I was talking to would be very irritated by other players trying to exploit the faults and bugs of the video–play–symbolic universe, other players become specialists in identifying these faults, in order to try to provoke unexpected events (such as walking through walls or accessing an uncoded space "outside" the game), as if they were trying to decomplete this Other.

Nevertheless, I should add that this code of conduct could be also seen to express a completely super-egoic morality, prohibiting any transgression of the symbolic Law encoded by the game designers and materialized in the video–play–symbolic space of the *gameplay*. As suggested by the young man's excessive gaming, the pleasure and amusement of the game was becoming increasingly less accessible to him and instead became transformed into a task and an obligation. The code of conduct prohibited even the slightest attempts at "playing" with the law by transgressing, exploiting or bypassing it, in order to derive pleasure from it.

A culture of digital objects?

For this adolescent, the pleasure of the game would, in fact, disappear once he had "mastered it." Knowledge was particularly invested for him and thus it was no surprise that even video games became a field in which he was trying to acquire a certain expertise. However, it was not just any knowledge, because in the history of gaming he was trying to rewrite, the 1990s – i.e., the decade of his birth – were an especially important period.

This attempt at historicizing this play object and, I assumed, in this way historicizing something of his own history in order to link it to a culture shared with others, was rather surprising. It really seemed that he was trying to use video games to rework a whole stretch of his own history – namely, against the judgment of his father. He disagreed with his father's opinion, which saw video games as something that made people violent or harmed their intelligence. His father embodied for him the opinion of adults in general – in other words, the dominant view which saw his gaming activities as solely harmful or dangerous.

Like many of his peers, this young man had a tendency to identify with the place of the martyr, the sacrificed. By depending on the play object as a true object with a history and an honorable status, he was defending himself against the discourse in which he was caught up and which tried to reduce him to a piece of rubbish.

Torn between two cultures, French and Algerian, the young man thus became invested in the so-called digital culture[28] as a place that would allow him to both differentiate himself from and oppose his father, who was sometimes violent towards his mother.[29] Video games also made it possible to imagine a career – for example, becoming a game designer or a game tester. Thanks to them, he could invest in other ideal figures such as the creators of the games he enjoyed. This digital culture offered ideals that could initiate different processes of sublimation.

Man, machine and . . . video games

Philosophers and scientists have often used "the animal" as an oppositional category to that of "man," trying to identify "a human nature" by contrasting it to another, even more "natural" nature, embodied by the animal. Technological progress has brought with it a class of machines, which have become increasingly more important in both our daily lives and in the questions of "human nature": the robots. One of the questions (which we find abundantly represented in science fiction) is thus of the relationship(s) we might have with this type of machine. It seems important to realize that we already have technological frameworks that engage our subjectivities, that modify and discipline them just as much as they engage our bodies; these experiences can already give us some hints as to the answer to this question. These frameworks are – video games.

Serge Tisseron is one of the rare psychoanalysts to become interested in the future of our relationships with these surprising machines – the robots – and he rightly draws a link between this relationship and the one we already have with video games.[30] Video games offer us experience of a relationship with a machine and with artificial intelligence, which are ultimately close to those we could form with a robot.[31] This relationship between man and machine has a long history, including, following the invention of the universal machine by Alan Turing, the popular metaphor of the cyborg.

External observers who do not enjoy playing video games often ask: "But after all, what's it for?" Why does one learn to use a joystick, decrypt all these rules and try to make progress through the game, sometimes having to exert great effort? The answer is: perhaps for nothing . . . unless it is the gratuitous spending of *jouissance* that drives us to act in order to exist, in the gaze of an Other.[32] The pleasure experienced by some players could thus be found in the fact of fulfilling this function for the Other-machine. In other words, faced with the demand that is pre-planned and generally expressed by the machine in the most explicit terms possible, the player tries to decrypt and satisfy the program by meeting the prescribed objectives. This produces narcissistic pleasure, a kind of *jouissance* correlated with the satisfaction of the machine's demand. In online games, this narcissistic pleasure is linked to the rank obtained, to notoriety, and so on. Hence the development of the esport scene.[33]

It seems important to me that this supposed demand of the machine excludes all sexuality, anything to do with the drive, contrary to all the Others that the child or adolescent has to deal with. The persons who care for a child indeed have a sexuality of their own and the latter permeates any demand they make of the child or the adolescent. Following Laplanche's argument, we could add that this is what forces the subject, having reached adulthood, "to translate" all the signifiers that remained incomprehensible to him as a child.

Excessive gaming

In some situations, the video game therefore represents a way of attaching oneself to an Other, whom we are simultaneously trying to bring into existence, in order to ensure, in turn, our own existence. If the machine becomes the only Other and there are no longer any adults or peers, it can be a reason to worry. In the case of excessive gaming, these attempts can thus be compulsive, just like in the case of this young man. He had a hard time doing without it or tolerating a relationship unmediated by the game object.

My interventions in this work, besides encouraging him to share his knowledge about video games, consisted in trying to create links between the history of games and the questions about his own origins, or between the "experience of the game" (an expression he often used) and "the experience of life with others." One day, we had a laugh together over the link that could be made between playing a video game and being able to hold one's own in a discussion, by using an interesting analogy: between producing a *combo*[34] in the game *Streetfighter* and making an argument in a discussion. From game performance to performative speech . . .

Excessive game playing could be considered as a particular modality of a relationship, where the subject is trying to create continuous *jouissance* for the object-machine, who has become the Other with the gaping mouth, threatening to devour us. *Jouissance* is a state that abolishes the subject, a state beyond pleasure produced by the injunctions of the super-ego, which constantly commands satisfaction and pleasure yet precisely blocks our access to it and eventually plunges the subject into terrible guilt for not managing to reach it. On the other hand, pleasure as a relieving of tension helps us put the brakes on *jouissance*, which continues to increase tension. The excessive player loses the pleasure of playing, which instead becomes a frenetic activity, in the case of this particular young man of methodically trying to finish all the games from a specific publisher or perfectly master a particular game character. Going back to Žižek's argument about the interpassive subject, excessive gaming would thus paradoxically be a way of trying to relieve the super-egoic task of enjoying oneself by trying to displace this *jouissance* onto the machine (Žižek, 2004, pp. 32–49).[35]

The moment to conclude

The video game as a cultural object involves us in a relationship with the machine that is completely singular. This raises many questions: what happens to the subject when he connects with these machines during a game? What kinds of *jouissance* and pleasure can he derive from it? In what way would this eventually displace the subjectification of his body? But also, what possible formations of the unconscious could arise from this experience?

If we think of the consulting room as a place in which, through the meeting between two people, a certain cultural work can be carried out, could we say that the psychoanalyst can potentially play a role in the transformation of the subject's possible relationship with technology in general and with the digital technologies in particular, given that the question of video games and the digital world (especially regarding social media) is now part of our clinic.

Video games, previously reserved to a small community, are now part of our common culture, as both a practice and a cultural universe. Thus, in order to grasp the way they are used today, we must of course start listening closely to children and adolescents. Let us give the last word to Winnicott: "I am also in touch with children's own references to their own significant objects and techniques" (Winnicott, 1971, p. xii).

Notes

1. This is an extended version of an article previously published in 2012 under the title "Au croisement de l'imaginaire et du symbolique, le jeu vidéo" (Video games: between the imaginary and the symbolic) in the French journal *Enfances & Psy*, No. 56.
2. It is customary to remind the reader that the turnover of the gaming industry has now exceeded that of cinemas and represents one of the largest cultural industries today globally. In 2008, it represented nearly €33 billion (US$40 billion) in turnover, with the United States leading the way. The last five years have seen the player population grow considerably; while previously reserved to an audience of initiates, young and male, the industry's marketing now targets "anyone and everyone" while the use of these technologies is becoming more widespread, the number of gaming consoles is growing (PC, home console, portable console, mobile phone) and the designers offer innovative and more accessible game systems (such as Nintendo's Wii).
3. Read especially "Chapter 1: Play Studies" (13–14).
4. For an analysis of the mediatization of this psychopathological perspective, see Mauco (2008).
5. Also see Stora (2003).
6. On this subject, see the special issue of the journal *Adolescence*, 69 (2009), "Avatars et mondes virtuels."
7. I prefer to distinguish between the game character, who cannot be modified at the player's will, and the avatar, which is by definition the product of certain choices left to the player, in general at the beginning of the video game.
8. Translator's note: although I believe "rewriting" is the most apt translation, *refaire l'histoire* is perhaps more subtle because it leaves suspended the question of repetition and difference: "redoing" history, repeating it, but also remaking it.
9. Triclot reminds us that "the arcade game is based on a fundamental principle: for the player to be overwhelmed by the game" (Triclot, 2011, pp. 150–156). The video game *Tetris* is a wonderful example of this.
10. Remember Freud's argument in *The Ego and the Id*: "The ego is first and foremost a bodily ego; it is not merely a surface entity, but is itself the projection of a surface" (Freud, 1923, p. 25).
11. "By virtual self-empathy, the avatar therefore gives the player *a figuration of the duplicity of his ego's image*" (Tordo, 2012, p. 121).
12. Again, my intention here is not to defend video games. The video game industry already does a good job of that. Neither am I trying to take any moral position on cultural works as a clinician.
13. These consequences have already been studied as part of the research on the influence of other media such as television. On this subject, see Bègue and Terestchenko (2010).
14. See also the chapter "La machine intime ou l'écosystème hacker" in Triclot which examines precisely three different social environments: academia, where video games were born, the arcade where it becomes a phenomenon and finally the family living room, dominated today by the TV set.

15. "Video games tweak the calculation to produce a strange and unknown form: a calculation that produces a dream, a dream woven by calculation" (Triclot, 2011, p. 66).
16. Using Marion Milner's concept of the *pliable medium*, later adapted by René Roussillon, Yann Leroux and Guillaume Gillet develop this link with the "pliable digital object" on their blogs, available at: www.psyetgeek.com and http://psychologienumerique.wordpress.com
17. This is why I am interested in the possible links between what Winnicott calls *destructiveness* and the digital matter, through his model of the "use of the object." See: http://vincent-le-corre.fr/?p=883
18. We know from Freud that repetition has an important role to play in child's play and, from Lacan, that it is closely linked to the symbolic field.
19. The clinic of obsessional neurosis is a good example. The goal of the obsessional's actions is that precisely nothing new emerges. For a more detailed presentation of Žižek's project for a new critique of ideology, read, for example: Calan and Moati (2012).
20. "Desire crosses the signifying line, and what does it encounter at the level at which it crosses the signifier line? It encounters the Other. [. . .] I am not saying it encounters the Other as a person. It encounters it as the treasure trove of signifiers, as the locus of the code" (Lacan, 2017, p. 134). This notion of the big Other nevertheless continues to evolve over the years and the space available to us here would not do it justice.
21. For a detailed presentation of Lacan's elaboration of the formula in his seminar, see Le Gaufey (2009).
22. Translator's note: The references are from Žižek's 2003 article in the French journal *Actuel Marx*. For an English version of this essay, see Žižek (1998).
23. These notions are more fully developed in, for example, *The Sublime Object of Ideology*. One of the philosopher's aims is to establish a critique of present-day ideology, which drives individuals to constantly behave in such a way as to mask their passivity and total submission to the system in place. Activity is therefore substituted for the passivity born by the Other.
24. Frédéric Tordo also explores this in Tordo (2012).
25. The second level of symbolization of the player's action are related to the Other through the demands that the game's narrative places on the player. I will come back to this later. The third concerns the social dimension of video games.
26. A *mod* (from the English *modification*) is a new game space developed not by the game designer but by a "simple" player from the original game. These spaces are then shared in the online player community.
27. "The Universe has been thought out, there are clear rules and perhaps a plan. No catastrophe is purely accidental, no new object without interest, no encounter with a non-player character fortuitous [. . .] And if the fundamental question addressed to the Other is: 'What do you want from me?', in *WoW* the answer is obvious. [. . .] The world has an intention: good actions during the quest are rewarded, as if outlining a morality of the world" (Coulombe, 2010, pp. 104–105).
28. For a number of years there has been a growing interest in *retrogaming*, a commercial movement that nevertheless seems to express a certain self-reflection on the part of the gaming community as to their own practices, an awareness of the fact that the latter are part of a larger history that opens up to a cultural universe with its own reference frameworks.
29. Beyond this singular clinical situation, for some adolescents video games have become a privileged ground where they undergo this passage towards adulthood, due to the fact that it often remains closed to the parents. The subject of video games therefore fuels generational conflicts in the family and crystalizes many other issues. However, this could change once today's adolescents, who grew up with these digital objects themselves, become parents.
30. See, for example, Tisseron (2011, 2015).

31. With the important difference that robots have a body – in other words, they occupy a physical space, are affected by gravity, their body has a texture which can sometimes evoke, for example, a pet's fur.
32. Unless, of course, we are talking about online gaming, where things become more complicated due to the presence of other players.
33. See, for example, the "esports: International Olympic Committee considering esports for future Games" *BBC*, October 28, 2017, retrieved from: www.bbc.com/sport/olympics/41790148
34. *Combo* comes from the word *combination* and denotes a sequence of actions carried out in a video game to accomplish a "special move."
35. This idea should be further elaborated in terms of the video game ecosystem, especially regarding the difference between online and offline games.

References

Bègue, L. and Terestchenko, M. (2010). La télévision favorise-t-elle les comportements violents? De Tueurs-nés à La zone extrême. *Esprit*, 5: 44–64.

Brun, A. (2008). Images fictives violentes et thérapies d'enfants: obstacle ou support pour la symbolisation. In F. Houssier (ed.). *La violence de l'image*. Paris: Inpress. pp. 73–95.

Calan, R. and Moati, R. (2012). *Žížek, marxisme et psychanalyse*. Paris: Puf.

Coulombe, M. (2010). *Le monde sans fin des jeux vidéo*. Paris: Puf.

Cunningham, S., Englestätter, B. and Ward, M. (2011). Understanding the effects of violent video games on violent crime. *ZEW-Centre For European Economic Research*. Discussion paper. Unpublished.

Fournis, G., Nabhan-Abou, N., Gautier, L., et al. (2015). L'écran et le truand: influence des jeux vidéo violents sur le passage à l'acte criminel. *Annales Médico-Psychologiques*, 173(7): 574–578.

Freud, S. (1920). Beyond the pleasure principle. *The Standard Edition of the Complete Psychological Works of Sigmund Freud (S.E.)* XVIII. London: Hogarth Press. pp. 1–64.

——. (1923). *The Ego and the Id (S.E.)* XIX. London: Hogarth Press.

Grossman, D. and Degaetano G. (2014). *Stop Teaching Our Kids to Kill*. New York: Harmony.

Gutton, P. (2008). *Le génie adolescent*. Paris: Odile Jacob.

Lacan, J. (1988). *The Seminar of Jacques Lacan, Book II: The Ego in Freud's Theory*. New York: Norton.

——. (1998). *The Seminar of Jacques Lacan, Book XI: The Four Fundamental Concepts of Psychoanalysis (1964)*. New York: Norton.

——. (2005). *Écrits*. New York: Norton.

——. (2017). *The Seminar of Jacques Lacan, Book V: Formations of the Unconscious*. Cambridge: Polity Press.

Laplanche, J. (1987). *Nouveaux fondements pour la psychanalyse*. Paris: Puf.

Le Corre, V. and Latry, G. (2013). Notes pour une métapsychologie du jeu vidéo comme objet de médiation thérapeutique. In C. Sternis and E. Granier (eds.) *L'adolescent, entre marge, art et culture, une clinique des médiations en groupe*. Toulouse: Érès.

Le Gaufey, G. (2009). *C'est à quel sujet?* Paris: Epel.

Lesourd, S. (2004). Reconstruction narcissique du moi adolescent. *Figures de la psychanalyse*, 9(1): 25–34.

Mauco, O. (2008). La médiatisation des problématiques de la violence et de l'addiction aux jeux vidéo: fait divers, dépendance journalistique et pénurie d'approvisionnement en sources. *Quaderni*, 67: 19–31.

Rassial, J.-J. (1996). *L'adolescent et le psychanalyste*. Paris: Payot & Rivages.

Robert, P. (2011). J. C. R. Licklider et l'informatique de réseau(x): imaginaire, impensé ou pensée visionnaire. *Études de communication*, 36: 111–128.
Salanskis, J.-M. (2011). *Le monde du computationnel*. Paris: Les Belles Lettres.
Steinkoler, M. (2016). Tueries en milieu scolaire. *Savoirs et clinique*, 20(1): 53–63.
Stora, M. (2003). La marche dans l'image, une narration sensorielle. *La pratique du jeu vidéo: réalité ou virtualité?* Paris: L'Harmattan.
Tisseron, S. (2006). Les nouveaux enjeux du narcissisme. *Adolescence*, 57(3): 603–612.
Tisseron, S. et al. (2006). *L'enfant au risque du virtuel*. Paris: Dunod.
——. (2009). Jeux vidéo: entre nouvelle culture et séductions de la "dyade numérique". *Psychotropes*, 15(1): 21–40.
——. (2011). De l'animal numérique au robot de compagnie: quel avenir pour l'intersubjectivité? *Revue française de psychanalyse*, 75(1): 149–159.
——. (2015). *Le jour où mon robot m'aimera*. Paris: Albin Michel.
Tordo, F. (2012). Psychanalyse de l'action dans le jeu vidéo. *Adolescence*, 79: 119–132.
Triclot, M. (2011). *Philosophie des jeux vidéo*. Paris: Éditions Zones.
Virole, B. (2011). Exil, combat et mascarade. *La complexité de soi*. Orsay: Charielleditions.
Ward, M. (2011). Video games and crime. *Contemporary Economic Policy*, 29: 261–273.
Winnicott, D. W. (1971). *Playing and Reality*. London: Tavistock Publications.
——. (1974). Fear of breakdown. *International Review of Psycho-Analysis*, 1: 103–107.
Žížek, S. (1998). *The Interpassive Subject*. Lecture delivered at the Centre Georges Pompidou. Paris: Traverses.
——. (2003). Fétichisme et subjectivation interpassive. *Actuel Marx*, 34(2): 99–109.
——. (2009). *The Sublime Object of Ideology*. London: Verso.

8

VIOLENCE IN REPETITION

Martine Fourré

This chapter touches on two questions that are currently guiding my research and that stem from my psychoanalytic practice. I have lived for 40 years with teenagers who have suffered with drugs, alcohol, debility, hyperactivity, disorders of multiple behaviors including psychosis and schizophrenia. Violence cannot be reduced to a theoretical question of "acting out"; violence is constant in the relationship we have with at-risk adolescents. This violence is a sign of a desperate call for an impossible presence.

The first question concerns the very Lacanian assertion that the father is the sole metaphor of the mother's desire in the structuration of the subject. The concept of the father as only a function, a kind of equation without a living embodiment, might seem to release men – those men we call "dads," whether male or otherwise – from the responsibility of questioning their own *jouissance* in their encounter with the child. Indeed, when a child separates from his mother, he moves from infancy to childhood and adolescence via social representations and the social links. During this trajectory, the father is not only the one who is present, assisting the child in this separation, as a result of the mother's love; the father is also the one that the child waits for so that he can take his child's hand to go into the world, a world that is not the exclusive province of the mother. This second paternal function – i.e., the function of authorizing – has often been overlooked by many psychoanalytic schools and movements. Authorizing is a function that concerns learning about the world, of the opening to the world as such. This function is the one wherein the child calls for his father at the right place: the place that traditional occidental culture assigns the father to inhabit. This first question suggests that the form and structure of the *jouissance* of the person who occupies this position for the child must be considered. Even if this *jouissance* does not determine the structure of the subject – psychosis or neurosis – it does determine the ways of making do, or not, in the encounter with discourse and the world. Even when the father is an object of identification, he is something more than a screen; in symbolic occidental representations, he is the first to sustain a reading of sentiments and dreams, of the use of words and ideas, mainly about the "mother," as understanding and therefore as acceptable or not by his child and in the larger world. So, while he is an object of identification in the mother's love, he is also much more; he is the way to go beyond that screen, to go in the way of a truth encounter . . . with the subject by himself. At least, this is how I can formulate the question for now.

The second question concerns this social function held by fathers, to which both children and adults implicitly appeal when "dads" are precisely unable to sustain authority acting as semblance [*faire semblant*].[1] Dads are asked to do this at the point of the subject's entry into the world's discourses, where he becomes a subject, where words and the body are knotted together at the intersection of experience. He can experience himself in the encounter with others. Aside from this examination of paternal *jouissance* in holding this space, institutional violence has been the unfortunate response by those who, unbeknown to themselves, are losing their humanity in favor of theoretical and administrative certainties. Such certainties exclude all questions about the *jouissance* of power that is held by those who are asked to respond in this place. They forget that realities are constructed by human beings by way of their encounters – of which the world is a product rather than a possession. By the way, we should point out that in France, this question had been cast off by psychoanalysts, even foreclosed, anyway, it is a question regretfully left outside its walls.

Nevertheless, on this crossroads, "repetition" plays a central role, just as it does in the encounter demanded by the analysand. This is always first and foremost an encounter with oneself, with the stories and history in which each imaginary self came to appear and search further than the idea one has about oneself for answers to existential questions. Besides its insistent presence in the clinic, the institutional rejection of the very idea of repetition marks the space where psychoanalysis and medical, psychological, social and pedagogical care meet, as well as meet with daily life. My clinic as a "question about the encounter between the subject and the social link" leads me to consider multiple causes and encounters over several decades. These intersections are critical to psychoanalytic work. Today, where fundamentalist terror and lone wolf killers panic the planet, such connections and intersections must be better thought. It is this very function of belonging to the world that seems to have been foreclosed by many psychoanalysts who keep apart the patients speaking in their warm closed offices, often comforting their own theories on the one hand, and imagine the world on the other. I add, this being in the world concerns both the analysts as well as the patients who see them.

Something has to be made more precise here. As pertains to the use of psychoanalysis in society, there is a real difference between the Anglo-Saxon orientations, both English and American, and the Latin options, especially the French-Lacanian. The first group took reality as a point at which childhood or schizophrenic disorders could be stopped in the transference; the second group rejected any taking account of elements from so-called "realities" in the structuring of the subject.

Today, violence, let us not forget, when it does not come first in the process of the infant's individuation, comes secondarily with the Oedipal complex, where the father takes his place, inscribing himself, in potentially paranoiac, repetitive, receptive fantasy. The very process of the individuation of a child's thought depends on whether the father is able to partake in the world's discourses and human representations. In this sense, reality does not exist independently from any child, but is produced by the encounter between a subject and the one in the social link that this subject calls upon to go into the world.

Clinical questions

Maud Mannoni, the co-founder, with Robert Lefort, of the Bonneuil Experimental School, encountered this phenomenon in her work with children and adolescents. In her book *Un lieu pour vivre* (*A Place to Live*), she explains the difficulties inherent to caring for psychotic children. She shows that the phenomenon of repetition does not appear only in the classical analytic treatment of neurosis, but also arises in the space of the social link in psychosis. Educators and teachers find themselves struggling with the same difficulties as the analyst. They encounter the same "symptom" that was behind the parents' decision to bring their child to Bonneuil and that inexorably marks all of the child's relationships with others and the world. Whether we are dealing with psychosis, perversion or neurosis, this phenomenon, or symptom, despite the differences in structure, is present in every encounter. Everyone is concerned by it: the cook as much as the headmaster, the teacher as much as the doctor. To open it up, to put repetition to work and help the children find other ways of relating to others, the team invented their "*séjours de rupture.*"[2] They hope, by doing this, that children and parents will find a gap, a real one – a gap that interrupts the repetition, a gap of no answer, a gap for dream, a gap to desire. During this three-week period (which can be repeated if need be), the young patients would go somewhere else – and hence must live differently in that somewhere else: at a farm or a school, in someone's family, in the countryside, or even in England. This experience introduced a space, a real space of difference. In this way, Mannoni also stayed in contact with her friends: D. W. Winnicott, Ronald Laing and Fernand Deligny.

In the context of what was then the anti-psychiatry movement, my family and I received the first children manifesting behavioral and characterological problems, as described by the pre-DSM nomenclature. It is therefore hardly surprising that, having become part of this therapeutic relationship, I too soon discovered the *jouissance* of "repetition" and its clinical importance.

Working in this small family environment, I lived with these children through all they brought to the world's stage. When I began this work, I was surprised to find myself raising a hand to a child who had been battered, yelling at a mentally disabled child doing his homework, ladling extra soup into an anorexic's plate, running after the run-away or preaching moral lessons to a delinquent who was possibly high on drugs. "I want this to stop" was the desperate meaning of my reactions. "Who am I?" was the question that came back to me. My analysis later showed me that these initial responses had a precise connection, both imaginary and real, to my parents. In my encounter with these children, the first that I worked with, my responses endorsed, even before I could think about it as such, the figure of the paternal Other that I had known from my own childhood: the figure of the Other, who, in a certain way, also solidified my presence as a mother of my own children. My father, raised in the ideology of the "Belle époque," which presented the physical masculinity of the paterfamilias as having complete control over his wife and children, had effectively imposed on me, by force, the order of the world which he thought himself obliged to carry. When my eyes opened, I could not help but see that by doing so, he repeated the tantrums of his own father, following the modes of childrearing that my grandfather, at the end of the 19th century, was unable to conceive of in any other way. My first gestures as a professional were therefore purely reactive, spontaneous, unfiltered by thought. I would think about them only later. They were even more troubling, because the accusations of social services simply added to the complaints of our young residents: children beaten in their families complained that I was just as harsh, young girls who had been raped by their fathers would run away to reunite with their lovers and suffer rape once again, anorexics lacking an ideal would devour my home-cooked meals and then immediately throw up in the toilet, not putting on a single kilo. Who was I, then, in the mirrors of their lives, if not the emergence of certain engrams of my own life? If not a monster, imaginary or real, who regulated their lives, unbeknown to them and to myself?

Repetition in institutions, in caring for the other, is first of all our own repetition, the repetition of the caregiver. It is through its sensations, affects and distress that the other calls for us, that he gives us access to his person and his own repetitions. How can we distance ourselves from the weight of this unconscious material – his and ours – while at the same time producing an act of welcoming and caring, one that could be heard and accepted? The administrative and political trend has been to introduce procedures that should resolve and guarantee this possibility. My experience has nevertheless taught me that this "verbal framework" of today's culture, which relies on many different rules, is insufficient, inhabited by people who themselves have made peace or not made peace with their own repetitions. Moreover, today's "rule culture," if we can call it a culture, traps people in a perverse dilemma. On one hand, if people obey the rules exactly, they can never exist as a subject of a personal desire, except to cheat on the ideal to which they have voluntarily subjugated themselves. On the other hand, as a chameleon they exist for the joy of cheating the big Other. These out-of-place outlaws, these "hot-headed" "ADD" children are beyond demand, beyond binding speech, beyond structures, and will rally around their problems by demanding both the presence and absence of others who are always necessarily in default. With the new clinical expertise, they will be shipped as packages, "unclassified," traveling between prisons and hospitals, the judicial and psychiatric systems. What caused trauma is never able to arise anywhere and is rejected even before it is able to dock. Today, we see the paradox of the so-called juvenile justice who favors the technocratic management of objects at the expense of living subjects, and thus destroys the very foundation of the salutary act he promotes.

A conceptual problem

I therefore had to think of, remember and elaborate the question of "Who am I?" I had to assert, in and through my actions, that I was not one of those Thénardiers[3] who enjoy humiliating the young to perpetuate their own status as the caring adult. Indeed, a lofty theorization was by no means sufficient to give meaning to "who I was."

This problem had to be thought through, but I could not find the words to think it, because the question of the clinician's intentions in his act had been radically excluded from the professional corpus of the medico-social field, and therefore remained unconceptualized. The social act was understood as ad hoc, as appropriate if it applied the moral, psychological and administrative criteria as technical recipes, and was considered completely independent of the practitioner's personal involvement. If the child or user was not improving, the blame was put on the wrong choice of institution or technique, or indeed on the person himself, for having inadequately participated in the project.

This technical and regulatory screen inevitably produces effects, including suspending people forever in those same repetitions that these measures were supposed to prevent or change. Had I not questioned my position and my *jouissance* in having power over the child, would I too have kept repeating my own childhood, as if to confine the one of the child in my care? This is how, in any given country, certain subjects find themselves bound to repeat the very violence that led to their social confinement. They can thus inadvertently escape the aims of a system that has been built on these principles: having been judged inadequate, they endlessly repeat the parental abandonment, violence and/or hatred they suffered. This is important in thinking about the institutional space. Research such as Philippe Declerck's[4] work on homelessness reveal, the true scope of this phenomenon, which results from failing to take repetition into account. It casts light on the dependencies these frameworks aim to heal, which in some cases increase the social gravity of the risks produced by these repetitions.

This phenomenon is a global one – and can be seen as the effect of a "universalized" administrative approach to mental and psycho-social disorders. During a conference in New York City in early 2016, three interesting readings by four psychoanalysts (Swedish, American, German and Italian)[5] highlighted the escalation provoked by this ignorance, by looking at the history of three "lone wolf" killers: Andreas Lubitz, Adam Lanza and Anders Breivik (German Wings, Newtown, Norway).

Dr. Frank Lachmann analyzed these presentations by focusing on the following observation: what these "lone wolves" all have in common is that they were trying to find, in the eyes of others and the world, the absolute power and violence inherent to their own experience: the engrams of their childhood. Lachmann pointed out that while most work has tried to explain their violent action by looking at their chaotic and destructuring childhood, few researchers have paid attention to the fact that, as children, these individuals also tried to appeal to some other presence than the destructive madness they experienced in their own flesh. Yet whenever these terrifying acts are attributed to the Stockholm syndrome or to the identification with the sadistic enjoyment of the aggressor, there seems to be an assumption that the environment is completely without agency. Lachman writes about Lubitz: "He consulted 41 medical doctors, including psychiatrists and psychotherapists, 41 professionals. What is represented here? What is continually reinforced? [. . .] Apparently, Lubitz informed these professionals about his feelings. And in turn, he probably became increasingly hopeless as he encountered 41 failed experiences." Hopeless, homeless, drowned, wandering aimlessly . . . having found no more place in the world than they had been allowed in their own families.

One of the main roles of the therapeutic intervention is to take responsibility so that this repetition becomes thought. When words do not suffice, it can be worked through in dreams, in less dangerous acting out that becomes addressed to the analyst. Lachman's sobering analysis summarizes the situation of a welfare system based on an exclusively technocratic logic. The readings of each one of these tragic events reveal the sadistic grip of the family situation, the lack of safety and security and the extreme suffering of these children, all of whose traumatic experiences become the bedrock of their passage to the act.[6] It seems as though in these cases, the practitioners, like the suffering individuals themselves, were bound to endure these breakdowns in complete helplessness. Nobody, Lachman observes, thinks about the fact that a response, "a welcoming gesture" offered to these lost beings, could have brought them some peace, given that they were only able to articulate a call for help and an annihilation in an endlessly repeating relational violence. In fact, did they not expect to encounter, in society at large, people sufficiently present and human, sufficiently receptive and loving, with an affection and presence apt to transmit some humanity, who could alleviate their feelings of being crushed and isolated? In their relationship with these professionals, why are there so many repetitions–reproductions of the abandonment and meaninglessness of the subjects' prior family life?

Lachmann answers this question: they have moved towards violent action because they had not been heard, because nobody came to their help when they were "brutally let down" as children. Nobody came to occupy, in transference, the place of reception and support that could have allowed them to open and invent a more peaceful and nourishing relational world. While pointing out that such is the current state of our conceptual thinking, Lachmann nevertheless raises the issue of the responsibility of a system unable to help these subjects open up to the world; he demands that we ask ourselves why so many professionals continued to ignore these calls for help. They were calling for a limit, for someone or something to contain and refuse their violence. By relying on a single mode of behavioral analysis and arguing, in the name of science, they as practitioners claimed to have no part in it.

The fact is that because I was practicing in my own home, I could not avoid the affective relationship in the same way I may have been able to in an institution, and because I could not exclude it from the everyday reality I experienced with these children, I could not separate myself from these reproductions/repetitions, or from the transference that supported each child in the encounter with me. I was therefore forced to think about my position, to situate and "name" myself and my function with each child. I had to articulate and sustain "who I was" in the transference. I was not there as an analyst, the other sought by a subject looking for himself, but rather as the Social Other, to whom the child was appealing to resolve the interrelation he experienced as putting him at risk, while simultaneously projecting this danger onto me. To admit that this repetition, in the analytic sense of the term, was taking place was, of course, against the orthodoxy of that time. Nevertheless, Rosine and Robert Lefort, in their clinical acumen, were quick to recognize the pertinence of this issue in their Preface to my first book on the social space of care, *Les lieux d'accueil*: "The aim is then – and this is what the ethics of psychoanalysis is all about – is [*sic*] to make it possible for an act to sustain the subject in his division. But is this possible in the transference of everyday life?"

When considering this question, it appears we have to distinguish less between transference as part of the cure and those arising in daily life, because transferential projections are the basis of identificatory phenomena in every context. On the other hand, demands in transference are not all on the same level. Teenagers most often "call to an undifferentiated social Big Other"; they are not making a "demand to the other of psychoanalysis" to understand why their life is not as they imagine it. Those very requests make all the differences as to the form and content of the responses of the psychoanalyst and psychoanalysis.

The "imaginary undifferentiated social Big Other" is expected in alienation to separate the subject from his *jouissance* and from his possible enmeshment as the maternal phallus. It is opening the possibility of division. This may be the same as sustaining him in his division.

From imaginary stories to conceptualization

Literature has always depicted the traces and immemorial acts through which human beings help each other access their humanity. However, inversely, it also shows us, as Lachmann does, that a human being abandoned at birth can reproduce this abandonment as violence, untransformed by thought or speech, against those he meets or whom he loves in his own paradoxical way. This is the case of Jean-Baptiste Grenouille, the hero of Patrick Süskind's novel *Perfume*. Abandoned under a fish-gutter's table as a baby, Grenouille makes his life into a mission to find the right smell that can nourish him, yet the horrors he commits on his way reconstitute the foul smells of his birth. Less frightening than this kind of fiction and more common are the so-called "novels of education" depicting a coming-of-age story or an initiatory voyage. Their heroes, manifestly driven by their questions of "becoming a man," are confronted with various trials and tribulations, moving from the innocence of childhood to adulthood, the German *Bildungsroman* being a national genre of such literature. This theme recurs in many genres, literature, painting and cinema. Except for where the horror exceeds our understanding, as in the case of Grenouille, these works all stage – along their own paths and their historical context – an encounter with the Other, a kind of life tutor, who offers the subject the words, gestures, attitude and surprise that dislodge him from his false certainties and help him imagine a different kind of life. Thanks to this, he stops reproducing the traumatic Real or repeating the real signifiers of the paternal Other that have marked his life and, by virtue of being able to articulate them in another way – as opposed to enacting them through the repetition – this otherness opens him up to the infinite range of encounters with others and with the world that he had previously remained blind to. On this path, blindness is replaced by insight; there is Oedipus, at the moment of entering into language shared and spoken by human beings, into the exchanges that "make" human beings. Boris Cyrulnik calls it resilience – a kind of peace, the ability to forgive oneself.

If we take the time to reread and think about the multitude of stories of childhood and growing up that make up our literature and cinema, it is striking to see the degree to which the figure of the Other is present and sought so that the lost children too can find peace. It is therefore not true that the figure of a practitioner able to welcome and receive the likes of Jean-Baptiste Grenouille, Andreas Lubitz, Adam Lanza and Anders Breivik is absent. We do not have to invent such a person *ex nihilo*. They have always been there – finely drawn by our myths, stories and novels. However, in literature the presence of these guides [*passeurs*], specific to the symbolic register, remains on the level of a story; it is not theorized in psychoanalysis, because analysts do not often think of themselves as implicated the material lives of their patients.

In Christophe Barratier's film *The Chorus* (2004), we see the lives of two figures of this social Other, two opposing caricatures: Clément Mathieu, an unemployed music teacher, and Mr. Rachin, an autocratic headmaster. The former's enjoyment derives from his knowledge [*savoir*][7] of an object of transmission that he tries to share with children, not without certain artistic demands; the latter, who has no such object to share, wants to impose order for order's sake, and delights in the children's absolute obedience to the power he claims. The spectator easily understands who will help the children grow and think, guiding their steps towards a future more bright, human and alive than their present.

In literature and film, the figure of the practitioner able to receive the likes of Jean-Baptiste Grenouille, Andreas Lubitz, Adam Lanza and Anders Breivik is not absent. It has simply not yet assumed the outlines of a scientific discourse – that is, one with equations lacking any affective imagination that would allow a community intent on making use of it to transmit it and guarantee it. If we understood more about our own acts, the acts that make us human, rather than about others' illnesses, this figure could finally also exist, professionally. Practitioners would be able to share and account for their acts in society and even formulate and narrate "the skills that help us receive those who cannot be 'integrated' in life."[8]

A reversal, an opening

Thus, my work retraces the steps I had to take in order to think about this encounter, about the moment when a subject becomes able to make the *pas-sage*[9] that opens up the space of humanized relationships, inscribed in the symbolic of his mother tongue. This can gradually result in a "reversal" that is much more powerful than the bureaucratic attitude of controlling the other, an approach that has increasingly invaded the structures of our medico–psychological–social sphere. Each day, being present with these young people has simply made me realize that it is precisely because of my lack of control over their lives and repetitions that they can make use of the analytic situation. While we derive our knowledge of psychopathology from life – everyday or not – this reversal shows us that the repetitions and reproductions cease not due to our will, science or power of making them stop, but thanks to our resolutely human presence and the freedom we offer the subject to "govern" his own life, rather than wait to be coerced by the Other.

Literature also shows us the moments of decision that produce a separation between two beings, the beginning of their true encounter, true differences, where their lives are interwoven through a recognition that escapes them. They stop trying to escape and take on the responsibility for their unconscious repetitions. In *The Chorus*, *The King's Speech* or *Catch Me if You Can*, the filmmakers follow the movements of reluctance and decision between adults and children, between those who are on a journey and those who help them complete it. The turning point occurs when the repetition changes its step. In the last film, by Stephen Spielberg, the young con-artist Frank (Leonardo di Caprio) travels around the world, posing as an airline pilot, a doctor, a teacher. The story begins with the lies of Frank's father, who is found out and humiliated by his wife; she then cheats on him and in turn lies about it to her son. The parents divorce. Does Frank begin to cheat – and eventually make his life into a series of con schemes – to save his father's honor in a cruel society, or does he do this in an attempt to keep his mother's affection? In any case, he becomes a likable and superior con-artist, able to imitate any signature, forge any contract or check, or pretend to be a member of any profession. He is eventually put on the FBI wanted list and pursued by an agent, Hanratty. He is arrested, tried and sentenced to 12 years in prison. The only person who visits him is Hanratty, bringing him comic books to read. What kind of relationship develops between them? One day, Hanratty shows him a check, asking for Frank's expertise to catch another forger. When Frank easily recognizes that the check is fake, Hanratty arranges for him to be freed and offers him a job, so that he can live out the rest of his sentence working for the fraud department. But over time, Frank grows bored with his new and wonderful life. Walking past a shop, he sees the airline pilot's uniform, the same one he had once worn himself. He buys it and decides to flee, but Hanratty catches him; he asks him about his life choices, about his relationships, his way of being in the world – in other words, he reminds him that he is free. Will he eventually come back, if nobody comes looking for him? And in fact, two days later Frank is back in the office. This time he makes the search for forgers [*faux-aires*] his true profession.

Based on my desire for a place that could truly welcome the subject in the modern and scientific world, my work has been moving from the imaginary stories that populate myths and religions towards a scientifically minded discourse that creates and sustains the social link today. Indeed, although these figures of passage and their legitimate guides have existed since time immemorial, nowadays in a society of consumption, exploitation and institutionalization, they have no legitimate space at their disposal. Nothing has explicitly replaced the places where people traditionally ask questions about what transcended them – spaces of religion or activism – about what was painful for them and what slowly made them become human before the gaze and presence of others. It is as if science – as fundamentally a knowledge about external objects, including people – made this impossible, technocratic and anonymous. I have therefore felt a strong need to produce a discourse about the act of being ethically present in society. We produce an act of welcoming and, by the same token, allow the transgenerational ties that transmit the discourses of "what it means to be human" and the "saying no" [*dire que non*] that gives texture to their transmission.

On one hand, there is objective knowledge: moral ideologies, technical and administrative applications to which the other is subject. In such an anonymous approach, no one is really responsible. This results in a violence that in turn produces more violence. On the other hand, a knowledge about the act poses objective knowledge and power as relational. This allows for the opportunity to question and exchange, through which both the guides and those guided enter into a social tie.

Who is this Other, who, one day, helped us access the human in ourselves, reopening the gaping hole of the infinite search for our own speech, asking the question of what it means "to be – human – or not"?

Spielberg's film gives us the first clue: it is the Other's inability, both in society and in analytic treatment, to legislate what is human and what forms humanity may take socially as well as individually. It is the Other's presence and his acceptance of what he can neither assume nor give to us. The lack in the Other and of the Other himself collapses the illusion of power that is fetishistically held onto by those who cling to objectified knowledge; it opens up desire for a different kind of knowledge [*savoir*], creating a space of possibility for each subject.

Now, let us summarize what the clinic teaches us. The subject's point of entrance into society is the moment, the space, where his questions cannot avoid an encounter with the Real and with the father's *jouissance*. This encounter, this interlocution, cannot be separated from the person of the father and his style of *jouissance* in how he exercises paternity. Likewise, alongside or, in some cases, instead of the father, those occupying important social positions (psychiatrists, psychoanalysts, social workers or caretakers) also must question their own *jouissance*, especially the *jouissance* they can take in that helping profession.

Does this entrance of the subject into society pose a question that has been rejected by psychoanalysts? And even by psychoanalysis as a theory? This properly Oedipal question is met with when the sexual drive meets the demands of life. This point of entrance has been rejected by many psychoanalysts who were blinded by the illusion of power that their science seemed to confer on their ideas about the very notion of reality. Yet the violence against those who cannot find this legitimate point of entry into their existence returns in the Real, as their boundless attacks against the spaces of the social link confirm that taking up a place in the world is foreclosed to them and outside their reach.

It is time to face up to the responsibilities that our own analyses have led us to recognize and rise to meet them by means of an act of transmission. It is the only way we can respond to the acts of violence of these lone terrorists and fanatics today. We must be willing to question the position of, and share the knowledge of the "psychoanalyst" beyond the space of the consulting room where it's isolated in a deceptive tranquility. It is time that the humane function of the analyst begins to work in the world, creating a space in which the question of "what it means to be human" can properly be transmitted. This is all the more urgently the case when science, whose discourse often includes psychoanalysis, refuses to know anything about these human questions.

Last but not least, in front of all the knowledge I have acquired during so many years of analytic work, I always wonder while taking care of those unclassified teenagers, whether my speech is generous enough and sufficiently open-minded to let them have a place in "my" life, and as a consequence to let them have a place in the social link, in their own lives. I always wonder whether my knowledge is something that I use as a splendid defence against those I pretend to take care of, or if my knowledge can actually offer a gift to them. The paradox is that nobody other than the subject concerned can ever answer, because if nothing happens in the subject's life story, this act – psychoanalytic or not – will not exist. But when some tragedy occurs, this act has failed, and so it has still not existed.

This psychoanalytic act is never visible, so its existence cannot be measured or substantiated, yet it gives a place to the unconscious. This indispensable, invisible part of humanity makes each man the caretaker of his neighbor, opening a space for the unconscious and for psychoanalysis in society. This place is foreclosed when the psychoanalytic act is not possible. The analyst is called upon by someone who is looking to become a subject of the tragedy of his childhood. This position allows individuals the dignity of an unconscious and the space of the Other.

Notes

1. Lacan, Seminar XVIII, "From a discourse that would not be a semblant." The semblant is at the level of the act, the closest to truth, thus of the real of the subject. It does not impose itself on others or on the world in a universal or totalitarian sense, because no word can stick to anything.
2. Translator's note: Literally "break holidays" or "break period" in the sense of breaking away from the children's usual everyday environment.
3. Translator's note: The Thénardiers are fictional characters of Victor Hugo's *Les Misérables*, where they represent a corrupt and abusive couple.
4. Declerck, P. (2011). *Les naufragés: avec les clochards de Paris*. Paris: Plon. Jean-Yves Barreyre (2014). *Eloge de l'insuffisance*. Toulouse: Érès. François Chobeaux (2011). *Les nomades du vide*. Paris: La Découverte; (2009) *Intervenir auprès des jeunes en errance*. Paris: La Découverte. Olivier Douville (2007). *De l'adolescence errante*. Nantes: Pleins Feux.
5. Klaus Hoffinan, The psychology of identification with the aggressor in individuals and societies; Siri Gullestad, Ideological destructiveness: a psychoanalytic perspective on the massacre of July 22, 2011 in Norway; Manya Steinkoler, School shootings: The case of Adam Lanza; Moderator: Marco Conci; Discussant: Frank Lachmann.
6. In French, *pas-sage* is a neologism. "Pas" means step, but also is part of the negation, *"ne pas"; "sage"* means wise. *Pas-sage* thus means a step towards wisdom while it also means "not" wise. In other words, there is something about being in the world that requires a non-knowledge or that is not at the level of knowledge. This is precisely what is lacking in the psychoanalyst who cannot engage with the reality of a severely suffering subject.
7. There is translation difficulty. In English, there is only one word: knowledge, which means "understanding of or information about a subject that you get by experience or study" (*Cambridge Dictionary*). In French, there are two words. Knowledge: "knowledge refers to a report of the thought of external reality and committed to the notion of truth as the univocity of thought and the thing" (*Encyclopædia Universalis*). Knowledge: Lacan stated in the field, this knowledge is unconscious knowledge, "savoir" of the psychoanalyst, "it does not stop not being written"; he is non-delegable and singular of each one.
8. Translator's note: The author uses the word *incasables*, a term often used by French social service professionals and field workers to designate an at-risk population of especially young people living "at the limit" of various welfare institutions and characterized by their multiple care needs as well as a history of presenting a challenge to subsequent integration efforts and care teams. See Barreyre, Jean-Yves, Fiacre, Patricia (2009). Parcours et situations de vie des jeunes dits "incasables." Une dimension nécessaire à la cohérence des interventions. *Informations sociales*, 156 (6): 80–90.
9. Translator's note: passage, *pas-sage* – "a wise step." Below, *faux-aires* ("false tunes") puns on *faussaires*, forgers.

References

Cyrulnik, B. (2008). *Autobiographie d'un épouvantail*. Paris: Odile Jacob.

Epstein, D. (2016). *Dérives adolescentes: de la délinquance au djihadisme*. Paris: Éditions Érès.

Fourré, M. (1989). *Les lieux d'accueil: espace social et éthique psychanalytique*. Introduction by Rosine and Robert Lefort. Nice: Z'éditions.

Mannoni, M. (1976). *Un lieu pour vivre*. Paris: Seuil.

Szpacenkopf, M. (2010). Maud Mannoni: apprendre une autre langue. *Figures de la psychanalyse*, 20(2): 163–176.

Vanier, A. (2017). "Maud Mannoni"; Lefort, Robert (2017) "L'antipsychiatrie". *Encyclopædia Universalis* (online).

9

THE VIOLENCE OF PSYCHIATRIC DIAGNOSIS

Patrick Landman

The violence of psychiatric diagnosis is correlated with its segregative dimension

The nosography of segregation

In recent decades, the nature of psychiatric diagnosis has evolved considerably. For a long time, its use had been restricted to psychiatric expertise that slowly elaborated a detailed nosography based on clinical observation. Clinical discussions motivated psychiatrists who were looking for the most refined semiological systems possible, thanks to a process of observation that was increasingly differentiated; however, these refinements had little effect on therapeutic procedures and most often they had no effect at all. This type of observation was also marked by the ideological prejudices of colonialism and racism. However, this period left us with an enormous corpus of teaching, some of which is very instructive and can occasionally still prove useful. Using the analogy of a dead language, we could say that the psychiatric diagnosis of that time was a kind of dead knowledge, far removed from any therapeutic efficacy. This diagnostic approach was discriminatory: it consisted of observing patients the way one observes, at the extreme, caged animals or plants, despite the humane intentions of many of its practitioners. This situation lasted until the arrival of psychotropic medication.

Psychotropic medication and anti-discrimination

Psychotropic drugs affect emotions, behavior, affects and moods; their use had a major impact on nosographic parameters. Since the 1960s, psychiatric nosography has become more and more pharmacologically induced, and mental pathologies have been redistributed and renamed based on the effects of drugs. For example, it was observed that antidepressants had an effect on acute anxiety, while sedatives worked on chronic anxieties – hence the new denomination of anxious states. From acute anxiety, panic attacks and chronic anxiety, we moved on to the generalized anxiety disorder. The emphasis is on symptoms, which are targeted by medication, rather than on patient experience or context. Although the arrival of psychotropic medication should be hailed as definite progress, it has also led to a type of dehumanization; the pharmaco-induced diagnosis could do away with listening to patients' speech, their experience, in favour of a medical-type semiology in which a purely formal meaning is attributed to the symptom reduced to a sign, and where we only pay attention to the symptom's formal envelope. The generalized use of psychotropic drugs has had many different consequences, but its impact on the discrimination of patients is more nuanced. On one hand, these drugs liberated the most severely affected patients and gave them a certain autonomy, helped them remain part of society and retain contact with others. No matter what we say, the "chemical straitjacket" cannot be compared to its physical predecessor. For patients who are less or little affected, psychotropic drugs have had a specific consequence: they have cut the individual from his symptom. The psychic symptom that is the target of medication is exteriorized by the diagnosis, in the sense that the knowledge is on the side of the doctor and the meaning of the symptom is reduced to a sign used for prescription. Some patients consider that the prescription of psychotropic medication is devaluing, and no matter how good or bad their arguments are, this feeling must be taken into account. Psychotropic drugs create a feeling of alienation; the patients no longer feel they have control over their psyche. This feeling can be transitory or it can last even after the return to normalcy. Sometimes they are relieved of their anxiety, their feelings of depression, their difficult emotions, but at the same time they feel dispossessed and have the idea that prescription is a tool of discrimination that is being reserved for those patients who cannot rely on speech or psychotherapy alone, because they are "too ill" or seen as such by the diagnostic approach. Thus, medication facilitates selection between those patients who need chemical aid and those who do not. The art of the physician, the psychoanalyst or psychotherapist can be used to counter this idea or help elaborate it, but the prescriptions of psychotropic drugs nevertheless act to separate us from the subject's speech and our listening to it. This separation can result in a feeling of depersonalization sometimes associated with an idea of discrimination that can become a narrative of devaluation and damage self-esteem. Taking medication is associated with a psychiatric diagnosis that serves to medicalize psychic states. The illness that the person taking medication allegedly suffers from becomes "objective." For example, the subject is suffering from an illness called "depression" and the doctor administers a drug called "antidepressant." In many cases, this does not correspond to any clinical reality or experience, or indeed to the real effect of the medication. It is a medical maneuver, a charade that works in some cases but often leaves behind a "remainder." The medicalized patient feels impotent and lost. He has not been able to speak or be listened to, as he would have hoped, in order to find a meaning for his experience.

The 1980s paradigm change and its impact on the segregation of the mentally ill

The arrival of the American DSM-III, which has gradually come to dominate psychiatry globally, brought about a large-scale paradigm shift in the psychiatric field. A number of factors have contributed to making psychiatric diagnosis less segregative.

First of all, it promoted the idea that mental illnesses were reducible to brain diseases, that they were linked to a "chemical imbalance" that should be treated with medication. This argument benefited pharmaceutical companies. Under the influence of scientific and reductionist theories, the authors of DSM-III, and subsequently DSM-IV and DSM-V, believed that the discovery of biological markers, which could establish both a diagnosis and a prognosis, and indeed determine an exact cause, was imminent. However, if mental illnesses are simply brain diseases, we can assume that they are a disease just like any other. No one would think of discriminating against patients suffering from a cardiac disease or hepatitis, and therefore we should feel the same about a disease of the brain, which is, after all, an organ like any other. Some years ago, the Royal College of Psychiatrists, the professional body of psychiatrists in the United Kingdom, launched a campaign with precisely this theme: "A mental illness is an illness like any other." Recently, there has been a new campaign entitled "Only us," implying "Only us rather than us and them." The results were inconclusive, because the campaign was founded on the idea that the fear of madness is linked to the lack of explanation of its causes, when in reality this fear, a key reason for the segregation of the mentally ill, cannot be reduced to the ignorance of aetiology; it is anthropological or at least cultural, and these campaigns, the usefulness of which I do not contest in the least, are somewhat naive in this respect.

The second factor was the emergence of psychiatric users as stakeholders in the process of diagnosis. Prior to the 1980s, expertise was held by the clinician, the psychiatrist; the emergence of psychiatric users brought in a new expertise, the expertise of experience. The families of mentally ill children and former psychiatric patients came together to form associations that discussed and elaborated psychiatric classifications, that had things to say about pathologies and their denomination, which, they determined, could be seen as discriminatory. The fact that users have become high-level stakeholders is exemplary evidence of the democratic process. Of course, there are some perverse effects, because a psychiatric diagnosis gives access to rights to claim social benefits and services, as well as educational and financial help. The recent history of the DSM has shown that this access to rights resulted in some patient groups effectively lobbying for certain pathologies to be recognized and included in the classification.

It is a paradox, but for several decades we have been living in a period in which psychiatric diagnosis is something that is called for and reclaimed, rather than associated with a stigma. It allows the individual to "know" what he is suffering from, to learn to live with it, especially thanks to helpful peers who have gone through the same experience and practice mutual aid in user organizations. The professionalization of these is on the agenda and helps the therapeutic education of professionals, using the management of diabetes as their model.

Although psychiatric diagnosis can sometimes be claimed, not everyone accepts it. This non-acceptance is not only individual; it is shared by professionals or users that form what we call in a pejorative way, "Antipsychiatry movements." These movements, which have existed since the 1960s, were marked by a number of different great thinkers of madness, such as Basaglia or Szasz, both innovators and sectarians. They were often inspired by psychiatrists themselves. Two years ago, some psychiatrists launched, with strong arguments, a petition calling to abolish psychiatric diagnoses altogether.

What we see here are, in fact, two distinct ideological trends that reinforce each other: on one hand, the reduction of mental illness to a disabling brain pathology, which pushes towards the integration of psychiatric diagnosis in the medical field and thus the de facto elimination of "madness," the fear of which which would lead to incarceration and segregation. On the other hand, a vast movement rejecting the medicalization of madness, whose annual "Mad Pride" publicly reclaims the right to be different, to have a different way of being yet enjoy full political rights, or the right to neurodiversity.

And finally, a new conception, still incipient, of the psychiatric diagnosis founded on the idea of transdiagnostic factors, especially *internalization* (which is present in anxiety, depression and phobias) and *externalization* (present in the different ways of acting out and addictions), which in turn call for the redrafting of nosographic categories and diagnosis. These factors are key in determining the impact on socialization and the effects of discrimination. For the moment, there are not enough studies, but perhaps this is a heuristic approach.

Is the disappearance of psychiatry and diagnosis a solution to segregation?

Since its origins, psychiatry has been guilty of two original sins. The first is its supposed non-scientificity; the second is the fact of incarceration. For over 200 years, there have been regular calls to denounce these sins and act accordingly. I would quote Pinel's liberatory gesture, Freud's redefinition of the border between normality and madness, Szasz's abolition of the myth of mental illness, Tosquelles and his successors who humanized psychiatry through institutional psychotherapy, Basaglia's opening of the asylums, but also Laing and Cooper, who claimed that mental alienation was a form of social alienation that was to disappear through political liberation – and many others, including, of course, Foucault. The list is long, their thoughts very interesting, and their actions do not take the same direction but converge on a critique of psychiatry.

Somewhat schematically we could say that by reducing the thresholds of inclusions in the different pathologies, by adding a psychiatric dimension to ordinary affects and behaviors as well as inventing quixotic illnesses under the influence of pharmaceutical companies – the famous disease mongering – the DSM forces us to think that all normal individuals are mad, while the different anti-psychiatric movements instead allege that all mad people are, in fact, normal. Sounding a more cautious note, Freud said that all normal individuals have a bit of madness in them and that all mad people preserve a part of normality.

The critique of psychiatry is necessary, but will its probable and planned disappearance as a medical discipline and its replacement by a new neurology founded on neuroscientific advances and a new set of psycho-social care services, even if economically viable and politically feasible, reduce the segregation of psychiatric patients? I am not sure, but only the future will tell, because frankly how do we even imagine the disappearance of madness? It is impossible, given that madness is also linked to language, the social field and to liberty, to the political treatment of "*jouissance*." According to Lacan, it constitutes an unavoidable Real, containing a real core that cannot be reduced to the social or the political. The degree of democracy of a given society can also be measured by the way it treats its mentally ill.

We should not confuse the political struggle to "liberate" individuals from mental alienation, a struggle promoted in the 1970s and still today by certain forms of actions, and the anti-segregationist political struggle for the just, fair and humane treatment of individuals who suffer from mental pathologies, which can bring together both users and psychiatric professionals. The two struggles are complementary. In other words, the disappearance of psychiatry is not in itself a miracle solution to segregation.

References

Freud, S. (1909). Some general remarks on hysterical attacks. *The Standard Edition of the Complete Psychological Works of Sigmund Freud (S.E.)* IX. London: Hogarth Press. pp. 227–234.

—— (1924). *The Loss of Reality in Neurosis and Psychosis (S.E.)* XIX. London: Hogarth Press. pp. 181–188.

—— (1925). *Negation (S.E.)* XIX. London: Hogarth Press. pp. 233–240.

Hochmann, J. (2015). *Les antipsychiatries: une histoire*. Paris: Odile Jacob.

Lacan, J. (2001). Allocution sur les psychoses de l'enfant. *Autres écrits*. Paris: Seuil. pp. 361–371.

Landman, P. (2015). *Tous Hyperactifs*. Paris: Albin Michel.

10

HOW TO MEASURE WHAT

Notes on universals and particulars

Todd Dean

Some years back I was asked to do some pro bono work with war refugees. For various reasons, St. Louis had become a destination for refugees, and since the last several years had seen quite a few wars, there was a lot of work to be done. At first, I mostly conducted diagnostic assessments that were used for legal purposes, such as determining if someone had to learn English before applying for citizenship, or had a psychiatric diagnosis that might militate against being deported. Eventually, I worked for a clinical agency to do therapeutic work. I had been working as an analyst and psychiatrist off the bureaucratic grid, so to speak, for several years before then, and filling out forms and questionnaires as a way of documenting the need for treatment and its progress was a new experience for me, or at least one I hadn't had in a long time; rather, 20 years ago I had to do things like this, but nowhere near as much paperwork went into it then as now.

The most striking thing to me was the number of clinical assessment forms I was expected to fill out for every patient I saw. The most common of these were the "Mind over Mood" inventories for anxiety and depression.[1] In the agency I was working for, every clinician must do both the depression and the anxiety versions of the Mind over Mood inventory at the beginning of treatment, and then every three months, with every client. The only thing that mattered, the only evidence on which we could base our understanding, were the inventories. These consisted of a series of statements to which the client was to answer with a number from 0 to 3, meaning that the statement was true "not at all" or "occasionally" or "fairly often" or "most of the time."

I'd like to describe the beginning of treatment with one of these refugees: call him Ishmail. Three years before we met, he was charged with having committed a violent crime. The evidence against him is only circumstantial, he tells me. He swears he didn't do it. For three years, he has been waiting for his day in court. He refused a plea bargain that would have meant only a few months in jail, because he knew he was not guilty. Now, if convicted, he will be deported.

He was seeing me, he said, because, since the charges had been brought against him, he cannot stop thinking about his memories of the war.

He tells me he was only eight when the war began. He remembers fleeing through woods, looking for safe zones. "When you see certain things every day, you are not shocked. It wasn't normal, but if I saw it now, I'd take it much harder." He repeated this to me almost every time we met. He also told me, "You don't know anything." He meant about what he saw as a child, what it is like to have seen what he saw then. But he always worded it thus: "You don't know anything." I came to appreciate that there were ways in which it was true: I didn't know anything. For example, I wondered why Ishmail had never applied for US citizenship. His language skills and ability to learn were more than adequate. Had he received his citizenship, this legal case would at least not have such potentially dire consequences. It was a mystery. But, again, I was new to this work: I didn't know anything.

When I applied for the position of adjunct therapist with the agency, I was told, "Their symptoms always go away when they get what they need – disability, a green card, citizenship, social security . . ." It was a statement of fact. For the two previous years I had done diagnostic interviews and a case conference with another agency, and had heard similar things.

From the start, then, Ishmail would seem to be a classic case here: he hasn't come for help until after he is in trouble with the authorities. Where were all those symptoms before? What does it mean that his memories of the war only came back to him in the context of the charges he is facing? But for the purposes of the Mind over Mood inventories, the only real question is: who cares? The first statement in the MoM anxiety inventory is "Feeling nervous." For Ishmail, today, the answer is obviously "3": "Most of the time" he feels nervous. But getting this answer really told me nothing, even though it was all the agency wanted to know about his nervousness.

I mean it quite literally when I say that having answers to this series of questions tells us nothing about the subject, even though it does generate statistical data that the Department of Mental Health for my state will use to justify decisions regarding treatment. This is because each of the statements to which the client must respond in the inventory stands in isolation. The fact that Ishmail feels nervous most of the time tells us almost nothing about that nervousness; further, we are free to imagine all sorts of things about what is going on – e.g. since he had never exhibited nervousness, so far as anyone knew, until he was arrested for fighting in the parking lot of a bar, why wouldn't we assume he was just using a symptom to try to get more lenient treatment from the authorities? Whether he has the symptom or is malingering, the same answer applies. But this is not a problem limited to bureaucratic paperwork.

Another way to look at this issue: the questionnaire provides an algorithm – a formula for determining, in this case, the need for services – that precludes any further thought on the questions raised about what is going on in the subject. Algorithms have become the replacement for thinking in our world – not just in the Missouri Department of Mental Health. Foer (2017) refers to the development of this kind of decision-making process as "mechanical thinking," "a series of precise steps that can be followed mindlessly. This is different from equations, which have one correct result. Algorithms merely capture the process for solving a problem and say nothing about where those steps ultimately lead" (p. 67). He goes on: "The process of translation, from concept to procedure to code, is inherently reductive. Complex processes must be subdivided into a series of binary choices" (p. 68). We see this in the Mind over Mood inventories, series of statements that presume to be describing something – pathological emotional states, call them – in an entirely objective manner. But, as Foer notes, "even as an algorithm mindlessly implements its procedures – and even as it learns to see new patterns in the data – it reflects the minds of its creators, the motives of its trainers . . . Data . . . tells its interrogator what it wants to hear" (pp. 70, 71). But data doesn't do more than that: it says nothing about why Ishmail feels the way he does, or what the way he feels has to do with his experience. The entire field of mental health care, I would suggest, has become quite algorithmical. Equally bothersome, it leaves room for whatever prejudice the observer wishes to apply.

Consider Jeffrey Lieberman's personal history of psychiatry, *Shrinks: The Untold Story* (2016). Lieberman devotes a chapter to the phenomenon of PTSD, the DSM label most commonly applied to the war refugees I saw. This chapter shares the narrative structure of the book as a whole: it starts by describing how horribly people were treated before war neurosis was defined, then how it was treated by early psychoanalysts making the traumatized talk about their childhoods, then how a statistically informed approach to diagnosis made a more uniform picture of the diagnosis, and finally how neuroscience allowed us to see the pathophysiological basis of the condition. The important points are the universal factors: the symptoms, their relation to a particular traumatic event, and the brain mechanisms involved in the expression of those symptoms. But when it comes to particulars, Lieberman has nothing to say: thus, he does not address the question of whether a sort of classic analytic treatment was effective, even though in his description it sounds ridiculous, and in the two clinical examples he gives – his own case and that of a patient – he has nothing to say about the fact that his own symptoms appear to have been so mild as not to have required any treatment at all, while his patient, after what appears to have been very extensive treatment, ended up as a severe alcoholic, completely isolated and unable to function. The one exception to this is that he does comment on the fact that he did not develop PTSD after being robbed in his apartment by "two thugs" with a gun, but did when he dropped an air conditioner from a 15th-story apartment window. But this is an exception that I believe proves the rule. He talks about how the latter experience engaged "the dynamics of the amygdala-prefrontal cortex-hippocampus circuit" because both he and his patient felt a lack of "cognitive control" (Lieberman, 2016, p. 269). But this begs entirely the particular question, how did he feel in "cognitive control" when two strangers broke into his apartment and threatened to kill him if he didn't give them his money, but not when he dropped the air conditioner?

The explanation he gives – that he did not want the thugs to find his grandfather's Patek Phillippe watch (p. 241), and so was able to override his fear to at least act as though he were in control of the situation – implies a completely conscious capacity for self-control: where did *that* come from? At first glance, what occurred to me was that he was not personally responsible for the thugs breaking in, but he was completely responsible for dropping the air conditioner and harming anyone who might be in its path on the side walk, at least as he tells the story. This suggests that his anxiety was the result of guilt in the latter case, not overwhelming trauma. Alternatively, as has been described in the literature on PTSD often before (Zaretsky, 2016), the trauma of dropping the air conditioner was more severe because it was entirely a question of what he imagined might have happened, whereas the trauma of being robbed was physically real. But in either case, this would be bad for his argument, because PTSD as here described is a group of symptoms that is always produced in response to traumatic experience, without the influence of such factors as guilt and one's devotion to one's inheritance from one's grandfather, or the material reality of the trauma as opposed to the fantasy of what could have happened. In this, the DSM – and modern academic psychiatry in general – is completely unlike those ridiculous old analysts treating soldiers with war neurosis in classical analysis. The DSM is a group of algorithms that reveal what (psychiatric researchers say) is real.

The inventories, questionnaires and forms we were compelled to fill out at the agency, like Lieberman's discussion of post-traumatic anxiety, are supports for a way of thinking about how things can be understood, a method of demonstrating truth. The 19th-century American pragmatist philosopher Charles Sanders Peirce was critical of this type of reasoning, because in it, he tells us, there is an assumption "that it is logically impossible for the premises to be true while the conclusion is false" (Peirce, 1932, p. 274) – i.e., if we make an argument that can be shown to have a valid premise, at least on the face of it, then all internally consistent conclusions are, of necessity, true. Thus, in the case of the Mind over Mood inventories, the premise is driven home that a ranking of severity on a symptom checklist defines the problem the patient is having. Similarly, in Lieberman's description of the development of the diagnosis of PTSD, there can be no argument with the notion that a traumatic event can precipitate a stereotyped set of symptoms – it all appears very logical.

Peirce continues:

> I think it would be just to add that demonstrative reasoning further pretends:
>
> First, that its premises are logically possible, or at least that the class of propositions to which they are considered as belonging contains possibly true propositions; and,
>
> Second, that its conclusion is not logically necessary, or at least, that the class of propositions to which it is considered as belonging contains propositions not necessarily true.
>
> Ibid.

In other words, the reasoning behind the inventories or the DSM is objective and can be proven wrong – therefore, they cannot be inherently biased: they are based on reasonable premises from which we can ascertain the truth.

What Peirce is describing is, in fact, the basis for the reasoning behind all of psychological medicine today. One need only consider the "double-blind, placebo-controled study," the gold standard of biological psychiatry since the early 1980s. Nothing is more irrelevant to the current situation, where, as Robert Whitaker, among others, has noted, there are more and more prescriptions, coupled with more and more psychiatric disability. Where is the eradication of mental illness?

At the same time, the universal assumptions Peirce is describing do violence to the subject. Every individual is subject to discourse, and every discourse is, to at least some extent, particular to that subject. In Ishmail's case, there is the idea that if he is only symptomatic because he is in trouble, he must be malingering – the assumption that the director of the agency makes every time. But, if the subject observing his case does not make that assumption, other possible explanations immediately present themselves. To take the most obvious example, there is the possibility that the trauma of being accused of a crime that could have profound consequences – most notably, being sent back to the land where he saw things that would shock him today – could precipitate a recurrence of his anxiety.

I will return to Ishmail and Peirce, but another clinical example illustrates the issue of particulars and universals from a quite different angle.

Ibro told me through a translator as soon as he walked into my office that his most concerning symptom was his asthma. He said it began "last December 25." He had experienced a few symptoms before then, but on that day, almost a year ago, it became a severe and constant problem, for which he has been in treatment with an internist. Over time, however, there were other striking details about his asthma: he mentioned that his oldest brother had been asthmatic since Ibro was a child. Later, that this brother was the member of the family he had felt closest to all his life; they even looked more alike than any of the other six children in the family. But besides this, there was the fact that this brother was hospitalized for his asthma shortly before last December 25 – which brought to mind another problem: for some reason, Ibro can't make phone calls to relatives in Europe.

He remembers very clearly the first time he was unable to talk on the phone. He had fled the country when he realized that male Muslims were being killed. Nobody knew what was happening or why, nobody knew then that near where he worked one of the most notorious of the death camps was taking shape. He just knew that he had seen neighbors loaded onto the backs of flatbed trucks, never to be seen again. His wife and other family told him to leave quickly, because nobody was hurting women and children. But the first time he called, a neighbor told him they were in a concentration camp. His memory of that moment on the phone was very precise: he became mute, *breathless*. He could not speak at all for a long time. After that, he had to ask others to make phone calls for him. For several months, he had no idea what had happened with his family.

After he was reunited with them, he didn't notice any difficulty with the phone until he came to the States. The move itself was traumatic: their turn to leave came as his father was dying, and his siblings and extended family – all the people he had lived with his entire life – were also going away, all to different countries and cities. Nobody remained at home.

Once in the US, the fear of talking on the phone came back with a vengeance: now he could not talk to anyone in Europe – all those he had abandoned as his father was dying – ever. At the same time, he developed a new symptom: he would cry explosively for no reason he could discern. This happened often, especially during bad time – e.g., when he was laid off from a job, or when he learned about his oldest brother's hospitalization shortly before last December 25. It was because of this symptom that he became extremely socially isolated, fearing to be out among people lest he suddenly burst into tears again.

It was striking how Ibro experienced these symptoms, his shortness of breath and explosive tearfulness and fear of talking on the phone. These were all physical symptoms, like a fever. The fear of talking on the phone, like the other symptoms, always happened in a stereotypical way, and was never described or experienced as being particularly meaningful, despite the memories he associated to it. It was entirely disengaged from his life. In fact, he was very much surprised when I pointed out that he had told me the inability to talk on the phone began when he heard that his family was in a camp: he had never thought to connect this symptom with the horrible circumstance under which it had begun. He likewise never described his crying as being very emotional; instead, he experienced a series of physical sensations that concluded in an outburst of tears, which relieved his physical tension, but was embarrassing. The sequence of sensations that led to the crying was described as though it were a completely autonomous physical event, having nothing to do with him personally. It made no difference that these outbursts happened only in certain circumstances, such as when he saw a news program about women and children being mistreated, or when he was at a celebration by his countrymen. Of course, his shortness of breath was no different: he just happened to develop the symptom on a date associated with his oppressors' biggest holiday, right after his favourite sibling, an asthmatic, was hospitalized.

The responses to Ibro's Mind over Mood inventories was particularly interesting. He did feel nervous, but only about crying in public, never about a possible traumatic event. His most debilitating symptoms, the explosive crying that kept him from going out in public or being able to find work, and his fear of talking on the phone, weren't even addressed in the inventories. In fact, his scores on both the inventories were fairly low even when he was at his most symptomatic, even though he was, in fact, quite debilitated.

The course of his analysis also was interesting for how it related to the symptoms he was having. Over the course of only a few months of weekly meetings, he described becoming less afraid of being around other people and crying hardly at all, except when talking to me. The crying also became less stereotyped in its presentation: rather than being the outcome of a series of physiological sensations, it seemed to have more to do with his feelings about what was going on. Eventually he also began traveling to see other relatives around the country.

But arguably the most interesting outcome of his treatment had nothing to do with anything we had recognized as a symptom. One day after he had arrived at my office for a session, I received a call from the translator that she had had a flat tire coming to meet us. From that day forward, Ibro spoke English, and we never again used the translator. He immediately was able to speak more freely, of course; for me, it was great that I only had to wonder about two unconsciouses in the room. But it also spoke to another way in which he had been alienated from his own experience: like the crying and the asthma, his inability to speak the language of his less-than-ideal land of exile was very much related to his ambivalence about being there – an ambivalence that he was now able to speak to. But again, all three of these changes had only the most tangential relation to his MoM scores. How do you measure them?

So, does that mean we need better diagnostic criteria, better symptom inventories? After all, Lieberman says of the DSM-5 that it "would now be a 'living document' and revised iteratively like computer software" (p. 272). There could now be a continuously revised and updated list of symptom criteria for psychiatric diagnoses. Maybe "inability to speak the language of the country to which you were exiled" could be a criterion for PTSD in DSM-5.1?

Lacan, in his reading of Charles Sanders Peirce's paper on the pretensions of demonstrative reasoning, would appear to be disinclined to accept this view. For both Pierce and Lacan, "the difference between asserting and not-asserting the existence of the subject ought to be the distinction between Universals and Particulars . . . Universal propositions do not, while particular propositions do, imply the existence of their subjects" (Peirce, 1932, p. 280).

But a particular proposition is not simply a statement of fact as one would find on a symptom checklist. Rather, it is how the particular proposition gets used that matters: "it is not enough for a proposition to be stated at the level of the particular, to imply in any way the existence of the subject, except in the name of a signifying arrangement, namely, as effect of discourse" (Lacan, Seminar XV, February 7, 1968). In other words, whatever value for bookkeeping or population statistics diagnostic inventories and manuals may have, they are alienating for the subject, every time, because they are static and therefore precluded from discourse. Or, to paraphrase a precursor of Peirce and Lacan, Hegel: "This is abstract thinking: to see nothing in the trauma victim except the abstract fact that he is a trauma victim, and to annul all other human essence in him with this simple quality" (Hegel, 1808, p. 118).[2]

I met with Ishmail weekly for a few months before his work schedule became too demanding. He had to work to pay his defense attorney. Every month there was a continuance of his case, so every month he had to pay more. In any case, he told me after a handful of meetings that he felt better: he was sleeping now, less distressed by the nightmares, feeling more hopeful. "This has really helped," he said. "Before I talked to you, I was a 1; now, I'm up to a 3." One thing I realized when Ishmail told me this was that it came as a complete surprise to him that talking could be of any practical benefit at all: there is simply no context for a talking cure in his world, no reason to believe that verbalizing his thoughts to a stranger could have any effect worth the effort – all he could do with his emotions was rank them on a numerical scale of intensity, much as I had to do to satisfy the demands of my agency. That was a way of understanding the world that he could understand.

Some months later I received a text message: "Hey dr. dean its Ishmail well I went to trial and was found NOT QUITE." The last two words were all capitalized and followed by a smiling green android. Just to make sure I understood, I called. He couldn't believe it was finally over, he told me. He didn't feel anything but shock, even some days after he got the news. He said he just wanted me to know, and thanked me again for having talked to him when things were going so poorly.

After I hung up the phone I realized that still Ishmail's behavior could be said to fit the paradigm I had been given before I started working with the agency: nothing in the propositions used in his diagnosis could disprove the idea that he had only needed help until he got the legal remedy he sought, as the agency director had told me was the case: QED.

But this is only even possibly true from the perspective of the measures used – in this case, the symptom checklist. Thus, if Ishmail's problem is defined entirely by the expression of symptoms – as it is in this questionnaire – then the fact that his symptoms come and go when he gets into trouble with the law is rather suspect: how can "real" symptoms be distinguished from exaggeration or malingering? But the measures don't take anything else into account – they are entirely static measures of something, subjective life, that is not static at all. If that were valid, then either Ishmail really has these symptoms or not: he's either symptomatic or he's faking – there's nothing more to say about it. The same could be – and usually was – said of every one of the subjects I have interviewed through the agencies set up for the treatment of war refugees.

There are many details I came to understand about discourse for people like Ishmail. For one thing, in the former Yugoslavia, everybody knows a story about somebody who had been killed or imprisoned for talking too freely – so there is a cultural disinclination to be too open with strangers. There is also, and perhaps consequently, what I mentioned above: there is no expectation that talking could help with a problem of this sort, so one would only talk when under duress. Then there is the fact that there is an expectation, since just talking to somebody really can't help, that one gets some kind of material gain from working with a therapist – either a medicine or a letter to the court or to the social security office. It also was generally understood that, as an adolescent from central Europe put into an all-black high school in the inner city, Ishmail had no reason to expect that any American was paying particular attention to his situation: why should he work so hard to impress an American shrink? I have heard subsequently that Ishmail has continued to experience a lot of distress, but to my knowledge he has not tried to see another mental health professional, probably because he doesn't "need" anything.

To conclude, I would simply like to suggest that Ishmail's text message to me after he got out of court expresses everything that Peirce and Lacan went to such pains about: he is on trial, and he is NOT QUITE: like every other subject, his situation is inconclusive, always to be subjected to the vagaries of discourse. I'd like to see the Mind over Mood inventory that can capture that.

Notes

1. Available at: www.anxietyanddepressioncenter.com/tests/
2. "This is abstract thinking: to see nothing in the murderer except the abstract fact that he is a murderer, and to annul all other human essence in him with this simple quality."

References

Foer, F. (2017). *World Without Mind: The Existential Threat of Big Tech*. New York: Penguin.

Hegel, G. (1808/1966). Who thinks abstractly? In W. Kaufmann (ed.) *Hegel: Texts and Commentary*. New York: Anchor Books. pp. 113–118.

Lacan, J. (1967–1968). *Seminar XV: The Psychoanalytic Act*. Translated by C. Gallagher.

Lieberman, J. (2015). *Shrinks: The Untold Story*. New York: Little, Brown & Company.

Peirce, C. S. (1932). Pretensions of demonstrative reasoning. In *Collected Papers, Vol. 2*. Cambridge, MA: Harvard University Press.

Zaretsky, E. (2016). *Political Freud*. New York: Columbia University Press.

11

FROM VIOLENCE TO AGGRESSIVENESS

Guy Dana

What is a field?

1

If today's violence has made security into one of our society's most defended values, it is because it has become a social phenomenon imposing its criteria practically everywhere.

When we say violence, do we mean physical violence, a "necessary condition" according to the historian Jean-Claude Chesnais (1981, p. 436), or are we talking about subjective violence? Is it violence received or inflicted? Depending on the context, the discussion of violence can therefore clearly involve very different, indeed polysemic forms.

My first reaction to this question is therefore to bring it back to the field of psychopathology with the help of psychoanalysis, while also exploring the area of psychiatry. However, make no mistake: the word "violence" originates in the social field and pertains primarily to events and facts – in other words, it remains very far from the clinic. In this context, it has replaced other notions such as aggressiveness, a term arguably closer to the subject.

Violence is both a common utterance, the object of sociological study, and a behavior, a symptom of something hidden and unspoken. The media, whose powerful amplifying effects are key to the machinery of elections, are partially responsible for this logorrhoea, which it then becomes very hard to shift. The difficulty of subverting a vocabulary that is now also gaining ground in psychiatry means that the word violence is, in a sense, imported. This is one of the characteristics of our modernity, which, as I will discuss later, undermines transmission as one of the key functions of language.

In psychiatry, the notion of security has therefore grown in importance, paradoxically where the phenomena of violence had previously not been a major concern. It is also true that certain tragic events[1] in France have short-circuited clinical reflection and imposed new norms. The psychiatric community became, in a sense, overwhelmed by the political and societal discourse.

Our first task is therefore to understand the foundations of violence from the clinical perspective, from the point of view of the symptom, or institutional complexity; moreover, the notion of security has slightly too strong connotations of order, while we, on the contrary, must be concerned with a framework [*cadre*], which is something completely different.

In psychiatry, this framework might mean first a concern with space, primarily in the sense of psychic space. Freud's own teaching and research end with a peculiar note devoted to space: "Space may be the projection of the extension of the psychical apparatus. No other derivation is probable. Instead of Kant's *a priori* determinants of our psychical apparatus. Psyche is extended; knows nothing about it" (Freud, 1938, p. 299). In other words, the psyche must have made certain acquisitions in order not to follow or remain stuck to the words or sentences that trigger various drive phenomena, as we often see in the clinic of the psychoses. It is when these acquisitions are missing that there is no longer any space for associations to be developed, and violence erupts. We can illustrate this with a concrete example: marching has always been a form of non-violent protest, while conversations on Twitter, where space is restricted, can easily explode.

2

Now let's think about the opposite of violence: it seems to me that what counts is not in fact security, but reliability. Security is necessary, because it counteracts the impact of violence, but reliability can act to avoid violence itself. In our field, we are always trying to construct an addressee [*lieu d'adresse*] for speech (sometimes even resorting to a speech pact), regardless of our position – as doctors, nurses, psychologists or psychoanalysts. We could argue that the fewer such addressees exist, the more *jouissance* there is, and thus potentially more violence.

To grasp this notion of *jouissance*, which is not always easy to comprehend, I think we must turn to the clinic of the psychoses. François Tosquelles was the first to articulate, in his own terms, how to find our bearings with respect to the question of *jouissance*: "Our path leads," he said, "from foolery [*déconnage*][2] to knowledge, from the language of connotations and intonations to clear concepts." This is what upholds the originality of the analytic method, which, simply put, works to transform *jouissance* into knowledge – i.e., into awakening, a new understanding. We should also note that for Lacan, speaking is already a form of *jouissance*.

The opposite of violence is the possibility of psychic and even physical movement, which, if organized as a movement between different institutional spaces, can be beneficial in the treatment of the psychoses. I have been pursuing this idea for several years now: it consists in building a territory of work that could be rightfully called a "field."

Yes, but what is a field and how do we understand it?

The title of Lacan's first lecture at the Rome Congress in 1953, *The Field of Speech and Language in Psychoanalysis* (Lacan, 2006, pp. 197–268) already suggested this primary concern: the need for a field to think about psychoanalysis in its act. His basic argument was that the field of speech and language becomes a space where "it happens," which is what enables us to work. In other words, within the confines of a field things gradually take on meaning and signification, once the field has been defined. Conversely, the passage to the act [*passage à l'acte*] is a kind of exit from the scene, where speech and language are precisely the scene, the field that the passage to the act rejects.

I have therefore tried to construct a field, to overcome the duality of inside and outside, to avoid binary logic that always leads to conflict, and instead encourage a movement between several different places, where there can be an effect of *après-coup*, where understanding arises from movement and where the differential between one place and another is articulated as a language. Changing the perspective and putting patients in a situation of translation means that the language of each place and the types of transference it elicits are not the same. The word "field" indicates that all actors, places and teams will have certain effects; ultimately, the term designates the site of transference.

3

Having disappeared from the field of representation, while simultaneously delegated to so many different organizations and teams, the *subject of care* now espouses less sadistic modes of therapy. Winnicott emphasized that we should not retaliate against madness (1971, p. 2); instead, containing aggressiveness and giving it space without letting ourselves be destroyed by it is a necessary condition for the individuation of not only children and adolescents but also adults. Simply put, we should not aim for a cure that is one and indivisible, but let elaboration emerge from this peregrination from one place to another; let understanding and knowledge [*savoir*] appear as a kind of reading between the lines, in the interval between the spaces, including in psychosis.

I think that we must defend another idea of psychiatry than what is currently promoted as "mental health." In other words, we do not want to become, to use a neologism coined by Marcel Czermak, "healthymentalists" [*santémentalistes*][3] – who evaluate, using precisely defined criteria, the efficacy of a standardized cure across different care institutions, greatly relying on psychotropic drugs (Czermak, 2003, p. 2).

The system we are defending obviously does not aspire to meet these assessment criteria, but neither is it trying to undermine them. It simply turns away from them, because of their excessive emphasis on the anonymity of practice and the sacrosanct principle of traceability. What we are defending is the possibility of subjective changes that value each subject's enunciation; all these are psychic acquisitions that attenuate violence. What seems dangerous to me today – as well as being a symptom – is that both the management and psychiatrists now use the same language. This relative porousness of the psychiatric field to "management speak" seems very worrisome. Its techno-scientist discourse excludes and permanently negates the subject, leaving no room for play, not just in the sense of a possible shifting, but also the creative sense.

Lastly, the addressee, reliability, space and play are the four essential ingredients of a practice that constantly interrogates its own violence.

The word "violence," while being a *portmanteau*, also evokes the idea of a transgression, of crossing the limit. The term itself suggests a behavior and, as Jean Oury reminds us (1994, p. 139), we should first ask about the violence that preceded the one we are currently faced with: "What has been violated in order for there to be violence?" By trying to think, when confronted with violent behavior, about its causes, by situating it in a history and a causal relation, we introduce the category of a possible subject. Violence becomes inhabited. In a sense, there is an Other. This is a kind of regime shift and it now brings us to the question of aggressiveness, which will allow me to resume my argument.

From violence to aggressiveness

1

We are living in an age dominated by real-time and image-based information. Real-time information is detrimental to psychic elaboration; instead, it provokes a response, incites reactivity and snap reactions – and this is already violence. Images appeal to the sources of our narcissism, the specular image and its ravages, reaching the very foundations of our ego constitution. However, in cases where, for complex reasons of deprivation, the continuity of maternal care is broken off too early or this care is not "good enough" in Winnicott's sense – i.e., when the environment is not reliable and the child is confronted with an outside, more or less terrifying – in such cases, the seeds of violence have already been planted. The child then perceives his environment as incapable of protecting him from either external or internal dangers, and there will be violence, or at least the conditions for it to arise. As if the aggressiveness necessary to individuation could not reach its efficiency, due to the lack of protective layers and the holding environment. But then, what is aggressiveness? That is the question I would like to discuss now.

In the *Minutes* of the Vienna Psychoanalytic Society, in the beginning of last century, we read that on June 8, 1908 the members discussed the hypothesis of the "aggression drive." As part of the Society's Wednesday meetings, Adler presented to his colleagues – Federn, Hitschmann, Rank, Stekel and Wittels – a paper he subsequently published as *The Aggression Drive in Life and in the Neurosis* and where he argued for the drive's existence alongside other drives (Adler, 2002). However, the idea did not sit well with Freud, at least not initially: Adler was told that his argument ran the risk of over-sexualizing power, to the detriment of the very foundations of sexuality and the libido. For Freud at the time, aggressiveness was to be understood in light of the drive's purpose, its movement, including the quantitative factor; he criticized Adler for confounding the aggression drive with sadism, which he thought should be distinguished as a particular modality of aggression. However, the works of Sabina Spielrein, Otto Rank and Freud's own later shift, in 1920, made him change his position: the idea of a drive component linked to the destruction of the world and other living beings was born. The death drive can indeed be responsible for such destruction if, as Freud never stopped thinking, it helps reduce the internal tension and keep it as low as possible. In other words, we can attack the other simply to get some *peace!*

What we learn from the debate between Freud and Adler is that in humans, aggressiveness develops in a way that largely exceeds anything we see in the animal kingdom, where violent behavior is dictated solely by need. Consider what Freud writes on this topic in 1929. One's neighbor, he says,

> is for them not only a potential helper or sexual object, but also someone who tempts them to satisfy their aggressiveness on him, to exploit his capacity for work without compensation, to use him sexually without his consent, to seize his possessions, to humiliate him, to cause him pain, to torture and to kill him. *Homo homini lupus.* Who, in the face of all his experience of life and of history, will have the courage to dispute this assertion?
>
> (1930, p. 110)

Freud borrows this Roman adage from Baltasar Gracián (1651–1657), who quotes it from Plautus.

Based on this, my colleague François Ansermet writes:

> We are afraid of the wild beast, but violence is much more a human affair; not only of the other, the unknown and distant stranger, but also the one close to us, whom we know well, our fellow human being – ourselves. What we are most afraid of is inside us; the thing most feared and most savage is what constitutes us. What we cannot bear in the other is ourselves.
>
> (Ansermet et al., 2002, p. 17 (translated))

Indeed, as Dominique Miller points out:

> never before has violence been so present in the public square. It is now practically a part of our everyday life, no longer found only in rough neighbourhoods or situations of crisis, but also in our living rooms, classrooms and city council meetings. Whether it is the criminal racket of one boy by another, even younger; a gang-rape of a young girl by her peers; the child abuse committed by teachers or priests; the exploitation of women and children from communities abandoned to the mafia, or finally the kamikaze

> terrorists who defend radical Islam and the holy war, today we are faced with a new clinic, which psychoanalysis has something to say about.
>
> (2002 (translated))

For Lacan, "man's ferocity toward his neighbor (*semblable*) exceeds everything animals are capable of, and that carnivores themselves recoil in horror at the threat man poses to nature as a whole" (Lacan, 2002, p. 120). In his view, aggressiveness and violence are subjective facts, by no means instinctual. There is a real of our original state of distress, a dependence that lasts longer for humans than for animals. This helplessness feeds into the subjective and imaginary phenomena regarding the other, who simultaneously represents the source of invaluable help and the greatest persecutor. To put it simply, a kind of paranoiac knowledge is constructed very early on, making competition and ambivalence part of human relationships. The Mirror Stage accentuates two distinct phenomena: inclusion, which can be defined as being captivated by and alienated in the other's image through identification, but also the mutual exclusion we could articulate as: *it's me or you*. For Lacan, the foundations of the imaginary register therefore repose on the real of dependency, and we should bear in mind that while we do find inclusion in psychosis, mutual exclusion is missing, which can no doubt explain the strange passivity seen in psychotic patients, like a kind of flaw in the general paranoia.

2

Whether they stem from dependence or deprivation, the different phenomena of violence bring us back to the very core of the constitution of narcissism in infancy, where the *infans*, the child who does not yet speak, is extremely sensitive to the environment – i.e., to the language that holds him, to the presence of the helpful person, to the appropriate actions of this other whom Freud calls the *Nebenmench*, our fellow man, the other, the stranger. We could also consider that the first act of violence *is* the other and try to reverse the proposition, working with the idea of the good-enough mother or therapist (which for Winnicott were closely related) and organize things in such a way as to create a potential space. We will then have to deal with the torments or at least the difficulties of institutional care as an environment that can itself become hostile, where we are constantly trying to look for the appropriate gesture to contain this violence, particularly in our clinical units. This brings me a letter written by Artaud to Jean Paulhan:

> Rodez, February 27, 1919
>
> Dear friend,
>
> I believe that by now everyone has read enough of my texts, since I was hospitalised nine years ago, to realise that, judging from these writings and all my letters,
>
> I am not ill,

I have never been ill

And to remember that in the beginning, my internment was only a terrible police business that has been kept under wraps.

Recently Dr. Ferdiere has been talking to me about leaving this place, but only to go to a maison de santé in Paris.

But for nine years I have been moving from one doctor to another. Surely you can see that I have had more than enough of the atmosphere of both hospitals and maisons de santé. I'm asking you to do something so that I am at last set free, plain and simple. Never again do I want to hear any other doctor tell me, as they have: "Monsieur Artaud, I am here to correct [*redresser*] your poetry."

My poetry is my own business and a doctor, no more than a policeman, has no competence in the matter, be it poetry, theatre or art, and this is something that, for nine years, the doctors have never understood . . .

Antonin Artaud

Why take Artaud's situation as a starting point to discuss today's institutional questions linked to violence? Artaud himself says it very clearly: the violence is that they want to *correct his writing*. It is not the electroshocks, the straitjacket that was then still in use or the rough handling by the caregivers (remember that chlorpromazine – Largactil – was only released in 1953), even though each of these could indeed be seen as an expression of a certain institutional violence, on the condition that we are careful not to fall, as it frequently happens, into the imaginary trap of identifying with the victim.

What is painful is always linked to enunciation – in other words, it concerns the dimension of the subject. It is when damage happens on this level, through different forms of negation, that there is true suffering. Hence, it is not the violence of the treatments themselves, but the way in which they are applied or prescribed. Furthermore, sometimes there are clinical situations in which someone is truly delirious, hallucinating, or even deliberately provocative, to which the care team must respond, while trying to adapt their response, so that a symbolic inscription is produced, if possible via the same gesture. And sometimes, you need firm and immediate restraint. I would add that this response, even when it is particularly vigorous, will not be experienced as violent by the subject, even in situations where multiple people need to be involved and when the physical contact can at times be rough – on the contrary. Bodily contact is much preferable to the distant and cold prescription carried out in the name of medical science and what is supposedly the patient's best interest?

The decade following Artaud's death saw the birth of institutional psychotherapy, initiated, invented and supported by the stubborn genius of Tosquelles. At the same time, the notion of the "care collective" (*collectif soignant*) became very important; indeed, the concept of the collective is indispensable to counter the destructive subjective effects of certain patients, let alone violent acts. We could compare this to situations of combat, where the trauma can always be more easily contained for as long as group cohesion remains unperturbed. Soldiers in Vietnam only began to suffer from the symptoms of traumatic neurosis once the group had dispersed and disintegrated. It was then that the veterans had the idea of getting together to try to piece together their memories (the so-called *rap groups*). Indeed, the more isolated the memories, the more traumatic they became as an effect of *après-coup*. Restoring the care collective or supporting these kinds of groups among patients through therapeutic clubs is vital to being able to withstand violence, regardless of its conditions of emergence: the violence of the intensity of clinical work, the noisiness of psychosis, the constant demands of the drive, the excessive closeness to the unconscious, which sometimes means having to impose limits both as a group and as a collective. Yet isn't it precisely at the level of the collective that things have changed today?

3

What we therefore need to analyze are the reasons why the situation has deteriorated in this respect. It has to do primarily with a discourse that maintains a certain splitting and that we could broadly describe as techno-scientific. This discourse undermines the foundations of the collective and makes us more vulnerable to violence, because our threshold of tolerance for it is much lower. The outcome is often paradoxical: psychotropic drugs are highly effective and we could say that, overall, institutional violence has diminished, and yet, as Jean-Claude Chesnais points out, the less violence there is, the more sensitive we are to it.

How do we then revive the collective, weakened by the divisions that, only recently, would have been unimaginable in the daily lives of our services? True, according to Lacan's well-known formulation, there is no collective assemblage (*agencement*) of enunciation, which underscores an intrinsic difficulty faced by each and every collective. From this we may deduce that if such collective assemblage did exist, it would be in the name of a common ideal, an idea that could potentially be shared, a few fundamentals. I sometimes think that without the support of a theory of praxis, which can, of course, be falsified and subject to the test of its application, there can be no collective assemblage. Instead, we should speak about the assembling *of* the collective, a kind of collective positioning, like getting in formation for a dance. Here, we again find the necessary subversion of the sector, considered as a space where institutional signifiers and teams are arranged in such a way that when they are traversed by patients, each trajectory becomes meaningful. We could also say that the compliance of care is replaced by the singularity of each individual trajectory: a story or even a legend are written, which is often essential for separation to take place. We cannot disregard the challenges of this approach: there is a real of enunciation of each individual, which does not necessarily comply with the collective and, as Serge Leclaire argued, there is no collective other than an assemblage of resistances. However, to combat this tendency, which I nevertheless think can be resisted, we must generate or try to generate a desire to care (*désir soignant*) and support team identity based on a general principle that the differentiation of spaces helps promote. It seems vital to support this desire to care from multiple places, before the collective assemblage of resistances has taken hold – which can always happen – or despite it happening.

4

I have previously tried to describe these symptoms of modernity in more detail (Dana, 2001) and so I will only talk about two of them: fragmentation and transparency, in addition to traceability, which I have mentioned earlier.

Regarding fragmentation, it is not a new phenomenon, but it is on the rise; the use of the DSM (APA, 2013) is an illustration, also no longer new, of this fragmentation. As we all know now, the DSM was created with the sole aim of improving the efficiency of prescribing psychotropic medication. The problem is that there is no longer any narrative, no historical dimension, that this mode of grasping the real goes hand in hand with an impoverishment of the clinic and a form of tacit negation directly affecting *the subject function*. Taking history into account, making space for the effect of *après-coup*, identifying the role played by trauma, not limiting ourselves to the level of the enunciated, but constantly looking for truth in the enunciation – if DSM is any indication, all these principles now seem to be perfectly obsolete.

In this perspective, the unconscious seems completely absent from clinical reflection and already highlights what I consider a very dangerous consequence of this state of things: that we no longer work with psychic conflict, instead replacing it with a splitting [*clivage*] – ostensibly to arrange, classify and categorize, but still a splitting. This has not only didactic limitations, but often terrible consequences for the care teams. In fact, when the gaze is prevalent and we only focus on the symptom, the quality of listening suffers, because it is only guided by clinical signs, to the detriment of the subject, who to a certain extent remains incarcerated. Listening thus no longer remains at the limits of the unutterable, where a potential saying [*dire*] suffers from not being able to be spoken – although this is the only way for the subject and psychic conflict to be heard.

Unfortunately, in psychiatry these phenomena of fragmentation are also compounded by the application of the French law on the 35-hour working week.[4] Although less objectionable in other disciplines, in the very particular work of psychiatry these 35 hours are synonymous with interchangeability, which not only poses problems in the relationship with patients, but also increases fragmentation.

The other symptom of our modern time is the mantra of transparency, brandished everywhere as the quintessence of social relations, yet also containing a form of negation. It is clearly a way of negating the unconscious, by annulling the structural dimension of language as what enables human beings to construct an intimate space from a necessarily incomplete knowledge of themselves. Instead, the idea of transparency makes us believe that it is possible to say all and prevents us from breaking with the specular dimension, or at the very least it encourages totalizing relationships, creates or foments the relations of paranoiac exclusion I have previously described: *it's me or you*. We only have to remember that the notion of transparency comes from the *glasnost* of Gorbachev and the crumbling Soviet Union.

Conclusion

To conclude, I want to stress that it is impossible to function in a system that is not democratic. As Marcel Gauchet reminds us, democracy is the sole system able to put itself in question and thus an essential condition for the practice of psychiatry (see Laignel-Lavastine, 2002). Conversely, this symmetry is not absolute: the psychiatric act and the therapeutic act more generally have not much to do with democracy and in certain aspects are not democratic. In other words, that is not what it is about: the therapeutic act always involves a certain amount of violence, and Piera Aulagnier (2001) even spoke about the violence of interpretation. We could equally argue that any dent in the *jouissance* that the analytic discourse and the therapy profession are trying to bring down or convert into something else comprises a form of necessary violence against the subject.

However, how can we understand the idea, so dear to Winnicott, that *we should not retaliate against madness?* I think that we must go back to the notion of space, and primarily the psychic space the caregivers carry within themselves; this receptiveness and hospitality enabled by the *extended psyche* is the antithesis of the pseudo-scientific discourses that instead erode it by systematically looking for a match, by dividing when they want to evaluate and making it impossible to look for psychic conflict. In contrast, taking this conflict into account has an effect on violence and enables us to work on a kind of "thirdness" in the relation. This means that we do not take ourselves for the true addressee of, for example, delusional insults, but understand that we are a kind of forwarder able to relay and elaborate what is being heard. Today, the tendency is to immediately make a complaint, but despite the humiliation caregivers can sometimes face, this legal reflex is a recent development, a sign of the damage suffered by the collective, the return of binary functioning and an erosion of authority. In other words, Winnicott's comment should perhaps be understood in terms of individual reaction-formations: the idea would be to *resist* the tendency to retaliate. However, for Françoise Dolto, who thought that adulthood meant moving from demand to indulgence, or for 19th-century alienists who argued that *the paranoiac is not cured but renounces*, the idea of overcoming violence does not seem to take into consideration the dimension of the drive, the quantitative aspects of which did not escape Freud and continue to mark one of the limits of our art.

Notes

1. The murder of a nurse in Pau; the killing of a passerby in Grenoble.
2. Translator's note: *screwing around, bullshitting* . . . there is probably no satisfactory way of translating the French vulgarism *déconnage*, or the verb *déconner*, meaning to do or say

something idiotic [*une connerie*]; the etymological root of these expressions [*con*] is clear enough, perhaps the important thing here is the idea of acting or speaking without reflection, which psychoanalysis helps us move away from, towards *savoir*.
3. The pun here is on "santé," health and sentiment.
4. The legal duration of the working week, a controversial French law adopted in 2000.

References

Adler, A. (2002). The aggression drive in life and in the neurosis (1908). In H. T. Stein (ed.), *The Collected Clinical Works of Alfred Adler, Volume 2*. Bellingham, WA: Alfred Adler Institute. pp. 62–68.

American Psychiatric Association. (2013). *Diagnostic and Statistical Manual of Mental Disorders* (5th edn.). Arlington, VA: American Psychiatric Association.

Ansermet, F., Halfon, O., Laget, J., et al. (2002). *Sens et non-sens de la violence*. Paris: PUF.

Aulagnier, P. (2001). *The Violence of Interpretation*. Translated by Alan Sheridan. Hove: Routledge.

Chesnais, J.-C. (1981). *Histoire de la violence. Les hommes et l'histoire*. Paris: Robert Laffont.

Czermak, M. (2003). Éditorial. *Journal français de psychiatrie*, 19(2): 2.

Dana, G. (2001). L'éveil du symptôme et les formes actuelles du malaise. *Che Vuoi?* 16: 89–102.

Freud, S. (1930). *Civilization and Its Discontents. The Standard Edition of the Complete Psychological Works of Sigmund Freud (S.E.)* XXI. London: Hogarth Press. pp. 57–146.

——. (1938). *Findings, Ideas, Problems. (S.E.)* XXIII. London: Hogarth Press. pp. 299–300.

Gracián, L. (1681). *The Critick*. Translated by Paul Rycaut. London: T. N. for Henry Brome at the Gun in St. Paul's Church-Yard.

Lacan, J. (1950/2002). A theoretical introduction to the functions of psychoanalysis in criminology. In *Écrits*. Translated by B. Fink. New York: W. W. Norton. pp. 102–122.

——. (1953/2002). The field of speech and language in psychoanalysis. In *Écrits*. Translated by B. Fink. New York: W. W. Norton. pp. 197–268.

Laignel-Lavastine, A. (2002, November 21). Marcel Gauchet, au chevet de la démocratie. *Le Monde*.

Miller, D. (2002). *L'agressivité et la violence en psychanalyse?* Programme of the College Freudien. Retrieved August 20, 2017. Available at: http://collegefreudien.pagesperso-orange.fr/stages.htm

Oury, J. (1994). Violence et institution. In P. Baudry and C. Lagrange (eds.), *L'Institution, la violence et l'intervention sociale*. Vigneux: Matrice.

Winnicott, D. W. (1971). Introduction. *Therapeutic Consultations in Child Psychiatry*. The International Psycho-Analytical Library. London: Hogarth Press. pp. 1–11.

12

WHY THE ZOMBIES ATE MY NEIGHBORS

Whither ambivalence?

Carol Owens and Stephanie Swales

> If you bite and devour one another, take care that you are not consumed by one another.
>
> (Paul – 5:15)

In this chapter we examine the lineage of the zombie and zombie post-apocalyptic scenes in film in order to make the argument that they fulfill essential functions for the speaking being under the conditions of neoliberalism.[1] We claim that the inevitable tensions of ambivalence, as well as the experience of hainamoration[2] itself are increasingly foreclosed under neoliberalism and moreover take place alongside neoliberal enforcement of the Judeo-Christian injunction to love our neighbor. This paradoxical operation accordingly produces specific effects: the return of what is foreclosed finds expression in violent zombie massacres and also operates to condense on the figure of the zombie all our foreclosed ambivalence towards our neighbor. In consequence, we argue that in times of foreclosure of ambivalence, your neighbor as the zombie next door is more likely to want to eat you than love you.[3]

The return of the zombie

The hit TV series *The Walking Dead* is exemplary in its staging of the contemporary speaking being's relationship with the social bond. In the "post-apocalyptic" scene, aimless survivors torn from their habitats wander through desolate, deserted, social and urban spaces, streets are strewn with corpses, stores and public buildings are devastated and burnt out – and there are zombies everywhere. Commentators on the zombie film phenomenon claim by and large that the genre serves an ideological function – the zombie speaking to what is socially, politically, or even psychologically current during a given epoch, so that although the zombie *per se* doesn't speak, what the figure of the zombie speaks *to* is indeed worthy of our scrutiny (Saunders, 2012). And what emerges to be current is entirely caught up with the fears, anxieties and tensions of the time.

The question that mobilizes much contemporary zombie film research is how did an obscure monster rooted in Haitian mythology and depicted in black-and-white horror films stumble its way into the mass consciousness of today's popular culture (Davis, 1988; Ozog, 2013). The figure of the monster in general can be seen to have emerged at a specific moment in history. The historian W. Scott Poole has argued that what comes to be constituted as an American "monster" emerges out of the central anxieties and obsessions that have been a part of the American psyche from colonial times to the present, and from the structures and processes where those obsessions find historical expression (2011).

At one of its points of origin, and as Moon (2014) and others have observed, the zombie monster's emergence is bound up with representations of slavery and colonialism in Haiti. Mark Danner points out that the movement from slavery to republic in Haiti was not unambiguously welcomed by the world's "first independent republic" – the United States, which, despite its constitutional and revolutionary creed "that 'all men are created equal', looked upon these self-freed men with shock, contempt and fear" (2010). Indeed, for all the great Western trading powers of the day – much of whose wealth was built on the labor of enslaved Africans – Haiti stood for the representation of freedom taken too far and fear rose around the idea that such revolt might spread across the sea to the states.

William Seabrook's account of life on Haiti published as *The Magic Island* in 1929, with his stories of voodoo and zombies, was pivotal in the constitution of the characteristics of the zombie in the first feature-length film of the zombie genre in 1932. Victor Halperin's *White Zombie* premiered at a time when the US occupation of Haiti was in its 17th year. The polysemous constitution of the zombie monster is observable in the merging of the "working dead" Haitian slaves of Seabrook's accounts together with what was an increasingly everyday sight for 1930s America: the out of work, destitute worker. For many researchers of the genre, the American horror film boom of the 1930s is immediately tied to the economic crash of 1929 and fiscal hangover, along with its subsequent misery and destitution. The zombie monster of the 1930s is also, then, a carbon image of the out of work, destitute, unemployed worker shuffling along the streets of America in soup lines, representing what Russell has called "an economic zombification of terrifying proportions" (2005, p. 23).

From the 1930s through to the present day, the many mutations in the trajectory and in the figure of the zombie have attracted much academic scrutiny and comment – especially given the malleability of the zombie as signifier and as allegory – and indeed as befitting a phenomenon that can be interpreted as "saying something" about the human condition and the episteme of which it belongs.

In his twentieth seminar "Encore," Lacan makes the claim that love marks the shift or movement from one discourse, one version of the social link or bond, to another. In our view, the zombies represent the displaced and tattered remains of the social bond, what is left after the love has gone. In "Encore," Lacan introduces the neologism "hainamoration," or "hateloving," in place of the term "ambivalence" used by Freud to highlight the point where love reverses into hatred, where the semblable is transformed into something unbearable (1975, pp. 90, 91, 100). Unlike love, hatred does not depend upon a discourse – or speech – to support it, and the hatred Lacan speaks of in "Encore" is the hatred that springs forth from jealousy. Coining the term *jealouissance*, he glues this hatred to *jouissance*, a *jouissance* incarnated in the neighbor, the semblable (ibid.). We argue that what is represented in zombie apocalypse scenes of human end times is precisely this unbearable *jealouissance*, which finds expression in the most horrific, brutal, violent and abundant zombie killings – scenes that indicate the extent to which the speaking being cannot bear his (former – i.e., now dead) neighbor's mode of *jouissance*. In this sense, the zombie is a fall guy, a stand-in, for the semblable, and, as such, a substitute for the ambivalent figure of "the neighbor," the one who is there, too close for comfort.

In a post-lecture discussion at MIT in 2014, Noam Chomsky was asked his opinion on the American cultural preoccupation with zombies and the notion of a zombie apocalypse.[4] Chomsky argued that US fears of a kind of avenging colonized mobilizes a narrative switch that takes place in popular American myths in which "the oppressed" are "transformed" into oppressors. In white America's collective nightmare the zombie functions as the representative of the realized colonial object, proxy for the marginalized unseen, unwanted denizen, offering American audiences an opportunity to variously sublimate and/or displace what they find intolerable in the (Indian/black slave/Mexican) Other (King, 1981; Wolcott, 2014). As such, the zombie figure becomes a perfect sublimated symbol for what society finds unassimilable – famine, holocaust, plague, toxic waste, genetic mutilation, borderless chaos, racial warfare, urban riots, mindless consumerism, etc. (Thompson, 2015, p. 22). Zombie post-apocalyptic representations of the human condition can be interpreted therefore as figuring something of the tensions of ambivalence inherent in society otherwise inarticulable or ineffable, while nonetheless ineffectively preventing the acting out of those tensions and the correlative unbearable experiences of hainamoration.

Freud and zombies

In *Civilization and Its Discontents*, Freud examines the Judeo-Christian dictate "Love thy neighbor as thyself" (1930). He famously asserts that although people would prefer to view themselves as "gentle creatures who want to be loved," the truth they disavow is that they are also aggressive beings, such that:

> their neighbour is for them not only a potential helper or sexual object, but also someone who tempts them to satisfy their aggressiveness on him, to exploit his capacity for work without compensation, to use him sexually

> without his consent, to seize his possessions, to humiliate him, to cause him pain, to torture and to kill him.
>
> (1930, p. 111)

In a Hobbesian moment, men, Freud claimed, are wolves to each other. We argue that at this point in late capitalism under the invisible grasp of neoliberalist ideology, men and women are zombies to each other. In this, we follow virtuoso zombie film director Georgio Romero who, at the premiere of his 2006 *Land of the Dead*, said: "[T]oday the zombies are our neighbors." Here is Freud on zombies, or rather, neighbors:

> Not merely is this stranger in general unworthy of my love; I must confess that he has more claim to my hostility and even my hatred. He seems not to have the least trace of love for me and shows me not the slightest consideration. If it will do him any good he has no hesitation in injuring me, nor does he ask himself whether the amount of advantage he gains bears any proportion to the extent of the harm he does to me.
>
> (1930, p. 110)

More contemporaneously, zombie film researcher Moon (2014, p. 204) argues: "the zombie has become a general metaphor for the other, who threatens our peaceful lives, rapes our women, kills our fellow citizens, and threatens the freedom of our society."

Slavoj Žižek has commented at length on the enforcement of today's neoliberal tolerance making use of Freud and Lacan's insistence on the problematic nature of the basic Judeo-Christian injunction "love thy neighbor," fully bringing out the attendant obsessive fear of harassment that accompanies liberal tolerance. As he puts it: "the Other is just fine, but only insofar as his presence is not intrusive" (2008, p. 35). In place of the injunction: "Love thy neighbor as thyself," Žižek advocates a "Fear thy neighbor as thyself!" This is because:

> [A] neighbour is primarily a thing, a traumatic intruder, someone whose different way of life (or, rather, way of 'enjoyment' materialized in its social practices and rituals) disturbs us, throws the balance of our way of life off the rails, when it comes too close.
>
> (2016, p. 74)

In turn, this gives rise to an aggressive reaction, as noted by Freud and Lacan, that aims at getting rid of this disturbing intruder. In *Television*, Lacan comments on the "melting pot" that brings neighbors face-to-face with (their) *jouissance* and prophesizes the rise of racism as a "*jouissance* going off the track" contingent upon a "humanhysterianism" (*humanitairerie*) understanding of the "Other" as "underdeveloped" (Lacan, 1990[1973], pp. 32–33). Picking up this thread, Eric Laurent remarks that with "melting pot," Lacan is criticizing the twofold movement of colonialism and the will to normalize "he who has been displaced, the immigrant, in the name of all that is supposed to be for his own 'good' " (2014, p. 2). Racism is understood as the minimum condition for the possibility of an individual's identity at the level of *jouissance*. Tolerance of the Other, of our neighbor, would necessitate "leaving [the] Other to his own mode of *jouissance*," but if our orientation as individuals and as a society is structurally underpinned by rejecting the Other's *jouissance* and imposing our own on her/him, we are tied to racism. What Laurent calls the "shock of different forms of *jouissance*" splits the social bond apart (ibid.).

Sociologist Anne-Marie Fortier examines how under neoliberalism, new forms of multicultural intimacy are imagined in contemporary Britain (aka "social mixing"), and how they are invested with particular ideals of loving thy neighbor and feelings for the nation. Fortier makes the point that racial, ethnic and cultural relations are not only negotiated and "managed" in literal spatial locations, but also imagined – we would say, following Lacan in *Television*, fantasized – through specific emotional and ethical injunctions, such as "embracing the other" and loving thy neighbor. Moreover, these injunctions are imagined in the ambivalent spatial terms of obligations to, and dangers of, proximity – an ambivalence that is inflected with articulations of "race," class and gender. Obscuring these "differences" between the lived experiences of speaking beings leads to a flattening out of singularity under the "equalizing" ideologies of neoliberalist discourse; the conditions for speaking about and from the place of the particular quashed in the fantasy that no difference is too great to be embraced for its very difference. In fact, the more "difference," the more "diversity," that is visible in such imagined locations, the better. In psychoanalysis, on the other hand, "difference" and its place apart from the other is the touchstone by which the speaking subject testifies to their singularity, and by which the articulation of ambivalence and its potential working through for what is imagined, projected and demonized in the other, made at least immanent in potential.

Therefore, we argue that one consequence of the condensing of neoliberalist discourse onto the super-egoic injunction "Love thy neighbor" is that it creates the bizarre and often dangerous outcome of a redoubled imperative: in loving my neighbor as myself, there is absolutely no place for me to dispose of my inherent racism, chauvinism, etc. One can recall the old Charlie Brown cartoon where he has been playing Cowboys and Indians using his right hand as a make-believe pistol. A speech bubble appears – containing his mother or father's command: "Put the pistol away!" That's just it. There's no place to put the pistol away. The pistol is always already there. Psychologist B. Keith Payne has commented on the cognitive "weapons bias" in which individuals tend to misidentify non-violent objects (a hand, for example) as guns when they are held by people with darker skin. And when the pistol is actually there, as is common in the US in which there are currently more guns owned than citizens to own them, the gun is fantasized to protect loved ones from a statistically unlikely violent home invasion perpetrated by a black man. Here, ambivalence about the racially different neighbor justifies buying lethal weapons. It should not be surprising that whereas in 2000 only 35% of Gallup survey respondents said having a gun in the home made it safer, in 2014 – post-9/11 and post-recession – that figure rose significantly to 63% (Kohut, 2015). Despite the fact that gun violence has actually declined in the US since the 1990s and has reached a stable plateau over the past 15 years, after 9/11 US public perception of crime rates and household gun ownership both rose substantially (Kohut, ibid.). Owning a household gun, then, can be seen as an index of what US citizens think about their neighbors (Kahan & Braman, 2003). The injunction "love thy neighbor" is currently embedded in a discourse intended to support an ideology of liberty and equality for all, but the problem is that the notion of "fraternity" – that other term of the "social" contract – is basically unenforceable. While it is possible to legislate against inequality and absence of liberty, it has thus far, at least, been impossible to make people "love their neighbors" without also causing vitriolic and violent hatred.

The more we urge and are urged to extend the hand of loving neighborly friendship towards our culturally, racially different semblable, the more, it seems, we want to eat or blow his or her head off (to bring to life Paul's words in our opening quote). Disavowing this basic human tension – highlighted in racial violence nowadays – is at the same time a disavowal of the need for speaking beings to stage the tensions of ambivalence, and constitutive of a panic-producing frenzy of epic proportions around what may be articulated as fears of "difference." Ignoring this tension on one hand fosters a fake tolerance at best, and on the other hand the nurturing of the narcissism of small differences building up into larger scale underbelly racism and hate crimes. Žižek's well-rehearsed point about the obscene underbelly of unpermitted enjoyment propping up the law of justice, fair treatment and equality is also observable here: what neoliberalism ignores (*lets it be*) is that ambivalent tensions run riot in the schools, in the workplace and in organizations, increasingly so because today's citizen is exhorted to love his neighbor, his school friend, his workmate, more than ever before.

Millennial anxiety and ambivalence

Commenting on the zombie film trend from the year 2000 onward, Ozog (2013, p. i) argues that while the rise in popularity of zombie films is directly connected to "our fears and anxieties as a culture," the decade 2000–2010 was one of particularly heightened social fears and apocalyptic anxieties. This idea – unsurprisingly – finds full support among the zombie film researchers. The increase is linked to the major fears emergent from the first decade of the 21st century: Y2K bugs, the attack on the World Trade Center of 9/11, SARS and H1N1 viruses, pandemics, hurricanes, tsunamis, the global war on terror, collapses of financial and social orders, etc.

What is increasingly referred to as "millennial dread" is, according to Kirsten Thompson (2005), simply an extension of an American apocalyptic tradition which in cinema was first represented in the 1970s in science fiction and demonic horror films as an expression of cold-war anxiety, then gathered momentum via a turn to social conservatism in the 1980s, and gradually reached a hysterical peak in the 1990s in a cycle of horror, disaster and science-fiction films explicitly focused on the approaching millennium. After 9/11, this "dread" took new forms with anxieties about the rise of Islamic fundamentalism and terrorism from within (Thompson, 2005; Stewart, 2013, p. iii). As such, then, and as Thompson argues, "social anxieties, fears and ambivalence" about global catastrophe under the label of "apocalyptic dread" took explicit narrative form in the cinema of the late 1990s and early 21st century. In this way, the zombie and zombie apocalypse films of the new century are seen to articulate something of the ambivalence specific to our times. As Bishop (2009, p. 24) notes: "a post-9/11 audience cannot help but perceive the characteristics of zombie cinema through the filter of terrorist threats and apocalyptic reality."

In our research, we found another important trend in film representations of the zombie, and of zombie invasions or intrusions into the human field. To begin with, from its emergence in the film *White Zombie* of 1932 through to the 1980s, the zombie appears most often as a supernatural conjuring, a monster from beyond the grave, or from beyond this world. This suggested to us that "the undead" as the roused dead neighbor, conjured into this state via some supernatural mechanism, is the zombie materialized of the real as a kind of payback for humans' meddling with the laws of Nature or of God, or, to reference Žižek, as a sign of a disturbance in the symbolic (1992, p. 23).

We had a hypothesis, however, that after 9/11, zombie invasions would be caused by something pertaining to human warfare, to the conflict of speaking being with his living neighbor. Indeed, after 9/11, by far the greater number of zombie films feature the idea that becoming a zombie, or being invaded by swarms of zombies, is the result of mysterious viruses or plagues, of humans meddling with chemicals, sometimes in the development of chemical warfare toxins. The notion of being "infected" therefore features as a dominant theme, as well as the idea of not knowing if your neighbor is already infected. If you survive, you will not be alone; you will, in fact, be surrounded by all your (dead) hostile neighbors. In the words of the character Robert Neville from the film *I Am Legend*, in which he is the lone immune survivor of the mysterious plague that has transformed everyone on the planet into zombie monsters, "God didn't do this. We did." God and/or the supernatural don't cut the mustard any more when it comes to explaining global collapse or apocalyptic doom. Rather, in our contemporary forebodings, it is the abuse of science, power and even capital itself that presage the arrival of zombie plagues and devastations (Rasmussen, 1998, p. 41). In what Jorge Assef (2013) has referred to as an anthropomorphic plague, man becomes the pathogenic agent of his fellow man, a point we are emphasizing here, as it is in the morbid twist which transforms one's next-door neighbor into one's next-door zombie, that we see the "hypermodern decline of Hobbes's thinking" such that man is in our times a zombie to man. The contemporary zombie is the result of a constitutive disturbance in the human world rather than an intervention of the supernatural or spirit world. Whereas before 9/11 your worst enemy was a zombie from another dimension – underworld/grave/even outer space – post-9/11 your worst enemy is a zombie created by your fellow man – your very own neighbor.

The new figure of ambivalence – the suicide bomber who is your airline traveler neighbor, the gun-toting murderer who is your dancer neighbor at a nightclub – is the semblable who incarnates pure terror, whose act devastates entire human landscapes, and whose desire is caused by an object whose *jouissance* is incomprehensible to you, but not any less deadly to you for that. If pre-9/11 the foreclosure of ambivalence resulted in the return of the ambivalent figure as a "zombie" from another dimension, we could say, *the real*: post-9/11, the neoliberal disavowal of ambivalence has produced its perverse counterpart – the "zombie" from next door.

Off with their heads . . .

The BBC drama *The Tudors*, which ran for four seasons from 2007 to 2010, detailed each and every one of the executions King Henry VIII ordered. We believe that these gory details, no doubt accurately observed from the historical records, fascinate us in much the same way that zombie killings and massacres do. In the time of the Tudors, the conditions for staging the tensions of the king's ambivalence were legitimated and anchored as custom, ritual and tradition in the symbolic of the period: if you fell from the king's love to his hatred, it could only end badly. In our time (and in most of our places), the public execution has left the stage, notwithstanding the enactment of the death penalty in the presence of witnesses where that act is still practiced: we recognize, of course, that the conditions for staging ambivalence are not the same as they were for our blood-thirsty ancestors as the symbolic determinants of our age are different. On the other hand, most "millennials" know the best way to kill a zombie, how and when that should take place, and judging by the sheer volume of zombie films in production, our sense is that the appetite for a good execution has not diminished much. To be clear, our argument is *not* that we need an execution in order to purge ourselves of our hostile impulses, but rather that as the conditions for staging what we experience as the tensions of ambivalence themselves undergo change from epoch to epoch, the ways in which ambivalence is "expressed" also change. And there are many things about which we experience ambivalence. As Adam Phillips remarks: "[W]e are ambivalent [. . .] about anything and everything that matters to us; indeed, ambivalence is the way we recognize that someone or something has become significant to us" (Phillips, 2015, p. 87).

It was none other than Freud's uncle by marriage – the German philologist Jacob Bernays – whose groundbreaking study on Aristotle and catharsis is regarded as having "overturned the dominant moral reading of tragedy" (Billings and Leonard, 2015, p. 8). Bernays disagreed with the notion that catharsis entailed a purification of tragic emotions – a common misreading of Aristotle in his view –

claiming that such a misreading had turned the Aristotelian interpretation of tragedy into a "moral house of correction" (Bernays, 1970, p. 4). Rather, Bernays argued that the suffering Greek audiences observed on the Euripidean stage offered them an opportunity to share in what he called the suffering "in the face of a collapsing old world order" and a delicious "fear and shuddering at the prospect of a fast-approaching age" (Bernays, 1970, p. 46). Indeed, he further claimed that social life with its "never ending reversals" offered a ready supply of "cultural objects" that can create the conditions for the experience of cathartic disturbances, pinned as these objects are to cultural pressures and cultural shifts (Bernays, ibid.). This view, which examines a kind of cathartic frenzy in representations of moments of social change and unrest on stage in ancient Greece, links very well for us to the arguments that zombie film theorists articulate in relation to the rise of the zombie apocalypse film, finding in the zombie its function as a barometer of cultural change and social unrest, as well as indexing something of the fear and anxiety emerging from sociopolitical conflicts and tensions.

Do this in memory of me . . .

In *Totem and Taboo*, Freud mythologizes the origins of the social bond qua transformation of Oedipal ambivalence into Oedipal fraternal guilt, and we catch an important glimpse of the functioning of the totemic meal which allows for the staging of the tensions of ambivalence while at the same time reinforcing moral law. If the resulting effect on civilized society of the social contract to agree to uphold the prohibitions on (maternal) incest and (paternal) murder is a fraternal guilt predicated upon an identification with each other (and our neighbor and our other semblables), then according to the thesis outlined by Freud back in 1913, there is a commensurate requirement for a totemic meal every now and then to identify (with) and work through our emotional ambivalence(s).

In Freud's advancement of his theory of the social bond at this time, he finds much value in William Robertson Smith's research of 1889 put forward in his book *Religion of the Semites*. In particular, he is struck by Robertson Smith's hypothesis that the ceremony of the "totem meal" had formed an integral part of the totemic system (1913, p. 132). What interested Freud was the function of the act of fellowship immanent in the sacrificial feast in which was stressed "confirmation of fellowship and mutual social obligations" together with the ceremonial aspect of the occasion involving the slaughter and devoration of the sacrificial (totem) animal. In other words, the totem meal celebrates identification of each member of the clan with each other through precisely a collective transgression, as well as ritualizing the identification of each member with the totem. What is forbidden to the individual member is justified only through the participation of the entire clan. Afterwards, the slaughtered animal is "lamented and bewailed" and this is followed by festive rejoicing during which "every instinct is unfettered and there is license for every gratification" (p. 140). This aspect of the totem meal suggests to Freud that this is how we can understand festivals in general: since it is an opportunity for permitted (nay, mandated) excess, it betokens the feeling that is produced when prohibition is lifted. But in addition we can see how the "lamenting and bewailing" is – as part of the ritual – something akin to a staging of something essential, something that should not be forgotten. First, there is the tragedy, second there is the festival, or first a *slaughter*, then laughter.

By contrast, we argue that in our times our festivals do not adequately address the tensions of ambivalence. Rather, we see them functioning much more at the level of that which Lacan called the "*semblant*" (c.f. Grigg, 2007): we are simultaneously seduced and deceived by the spectacle of the carnivalesque aspects of the festival while failing to identify entirely (with) the "action" or "drama" at the heart of it. In his speech at the Occupy Wall Street protest in 2012, Žižek advised protesters not to fall for the *semblant* of the carnival, proclaiming that even though the "taboo" is broken, it is still possible to be seduced into inactivity:

> Don't fall in love [with yourselves,] with the nice time we are having here. Carnivals come cheap – the true test of their worth is what remains the day after, how our normal daily life will be changed. Fall in love with hard and patient work – we are the beginning, not the end. Our basic message is: the taboo is broken, we do not live in the best possible world, we are allowed and obliged even to think about alternatives.

Carnivals come cheaply in our times. Now we go on Facebook and Twitter in response to events such as violent shootings or abuses of power. The taboo is broken: as Žižek says, we can stage mass protests at the drop of a hat. Our discontents are "things" that go "viral" at incalculable speeds. News is never "new." The hypermodern technologies of capitalism ensure a constantly "updated" news-feed and its counterpart in the form of endless threads, blogs, vlogs, tweets, snapchats, instagrams and other digital bites. Is this the 21st-century version of the Greek Attic chorus, we wonder?

Frances Ferguson argues that for Aristotle, the Sophoclean chorus may be described as a group personality – with its own traditions, habits of thought and feeling, and mode of being. It exists, it perceives, and it depends on the main protagonists to invent and try out the details of the drama. It is the function of the chorus to mark the stages of the action and to perform the suffering and perceiving part of the tragic rhythm (2007, p. 8). In this way, the function of the Greek chorus in relation to the staging of the tragedy can be seen to have mobilized essential representations of the tensions of ambivalence. For Lacan, indeed the chorus is "the people who are moved," the ones who take care of your emotions (Lacan, 1999, p. 252). Greek drama scholar Lucy Jackson argues that modern audiences faced with the spectacle of the Greek chorus experience it as a challenge: it is not, Jackson emphasizes, because of an intellectual demand upon the audience, but rather because the chorus prompts the audience to be become involved in the action of the drama (Jackson, 2015).

We believe that it is possible to see something of the same psychical business in the work of the Greek chorus and in the totemic ritual as each offered opportunities for the catharsis of ambivalence. Ferguson claims that Sophocles's audience must have had as much appetite for the thrills and diversion as the crowds who – in our time – assemble for football games, music festivals, or Easter performances of *Saint Matthew's Passion* (ibid.: 6). Perhaps this is true, but the proper symbolic resonance that struck Aristotle with the Greeks and Freud with totemic tribal rituals is seldom at work in present-day spectacles. Instead, we have a perpetual motion industry of homogenized totems: in lieu, then, of some totem we can love to death, the subject is in danger of becoming her own kind of totemic pillar of narcissism.

In the absence of adequate cultural practices to stage the tensions of ambivalence, we believe that there are outcomes at the level of individual psychopathology and at the level of culture. One way to take the pulse of our ambivalence is to examine our ways of storytelling, our own myths, which nowadays are more likely to be framed as a TV show or as a movie than the more traditional version as "fairy tale," folk tale, or puppet show.

That's (not) the way to do it

> Gathering around the crimson booth on windy Morecambe Bay, the children fidget and squeal with excitement. The show is about to start. Up pops the red-nosed hunchback Mr. Punch to welcome his crowd, before embarking on 25 minutes of slapstick. The children become transfixed. The more he shakes the baby and the harder he beats the policeman, the more they howl with laughter and the louder the cheers. The level of violence is hardly within pre watershed guidelines, but even grown men find themselves giggling like schoolgirls.
>
> (Sophie de Rosée, *The Telegraph*, September 4, 2009)

At the time of writing, Punch, the chief protagonist from the Punch and Judy puppet theater show, celebrates 355 years of existence. The show is characterized by much fighting and killing. The story revolves around Punch, who variously fights with the devil or a crocodile, beats his nagging wife and defenestrates his baby: on completion of his various murderous acts, he cries out, "Now that's the way to do it!" Punch derives from the "Italian puppet play" so-called by Samuel Pepys. Commentaries on the genre of puppet theater agree that "Punch" arrived in England at a moment of great social upheaval. The country's recent brush with republicanism had gone spectacularly off the rails after its leader, the deeply puritanical Oliver Cromwell, turned England into a dead zone of no theater, no dancing, no sports – no fun (Rodriguez, 2013). With the abatement of Puritanism after Cromwell's death in 1658, artists and performing troupes from Europe began to arrive in England and the puppet "Pulcinella," the Italian clown character of the *commedia dell'arte* tradition, made his debut on the English stage. Through Anglicization, Pulcinella became "Punchinello" which eventually was shortened to "Punch."

Punch and Judy researcher Martin Leech describes the puppet show as a theatrical form whose roots were firmly embedded in the cultural and political upheavals of the 18th century, and explains the composition of the show as a response to the beginnings of the institutional repressions of a developing underclass (Leech, 1985). Leech's research suggests that the emerging triumvirate of the law, religion and marriage as forms of social control were manifest in the show as the Hangman, the Devil and Judy (c.f. Reeve, 2005, p. 17). Spectators could therefore identify with Punch as he variously fought off and/or murdered the causes of his prohibited desires, which were also their prohibited desires. There was – as such – the opportunity to witness the spectacle of their own ambivalent tensions vis-à-vis the Law, and the opportunity for a bit of cathartic action.

By the end of the 18th century, Punch had transformed from its original form as marionette into the glove puppet booth form, and by the early 19th century new features were introduced into the show while retaining many of the features of the original one, including his shrewish wife Judy, whom he regularly beat and killed, and his encounter with the Devil. Reeve observes that several of the original puppet characters came to be associated with and transformed into actual figures of the time. "Scaramouch" became "Clown Joey" after Joey Grimaldi; the "Hangman" came to be named after "Jack Ketch," the most famous hangman of the early 19th century; and the servant "N*****" or "Shallaballa" became "Jim Crow" after the very popular black-face music-hall character performed by T. D. Rice in the 1830s (Reeve, 2005, p. 50).

In Britain, Reeve remarks that the show has not been subject to the same kinds of intervention by national or exterior agencies with agendas that have shaped and transformed popular puppetry in some other countries (Reeve, ibid.). One of the reasons for this "resistance" to change, according to Clifford and King (2006, p. 338), is due to its ambivalent position embodying the wild aspects of British popular culture as "shifting, offensive and anarchic." However, an article from British newspaper *The Telegraph* on the occasion of Punch's 350th birthday commented that the themes of domestic violence, assaulting police and general anarchic behavior, together with some of the more offensive characters (including the hangman), have been phased out. Journalist de Rosée argues that political correctness is Mr. Punch's arch enemy, and that some British councils have attempted to ban the entire show. In 2004, one Women's Rape and Sexual Abuse Center attempted to instigate a ban on the basis that children were encouraged to laugh at a family whose relationship was based on violence, and in 2005, one of the local councils banned puppets of Saddam Hussein and Osama bin Laden, cast as the show's sausage-stealing villains (de Rosée, 2009). Indeed, individual "Punchmen" (the puppeteers of the Punch and Judy shows) remark that whereas they continue to use the Hangman in shows outside of Britain, they don't use that character in British performances.

From his disruptive debut in 16th-century England, which was welcomed and praised by Samuel Pepys, Punch has been hailed by great satirist Jonathan Swift in the 17th century, and commended by Charles Dickens in 1849 for his cathartic effects, which he cautioned would be spoiled by cleaning up his act and removing the violence from it. What is clear is that the 350-year history of Pulcinella, Punchinello, or Punch, from Italy to England, and his counterparts, and European and further-flung cousins – Kasperle in Germany and Austria, Polichinelle in France, Karakoz in Turkey, and Petrushka in Russia – has operated in order to represent and stage some of the tensions of the ambivalence experienced during these epochs and in these places. What is noted by the diverse commentators in this field is the disruptive, anarchic and cathartic effects produced in audiences.

What is most interesting, of course, is that accounts from the early 21st century of attempts to remove aspects and characters of the puppet show because of the harm they may cause to children or the offense they may cause to spectators is both, as we observe, extremely recent and to a certain extent resisted (however, what is *foreclosed* from the British show crops up in other places and in other countries). What is most brilliantly illustrated for us is the literal removal from the stage of certain parts of the action (Judy is less often killed now and often returns unharmed at the end of the show) and certain characters (the Hangman is removed altogether). According to most commentators of the art form, the Punch and Judy show offered ways for children and other spectators to identify with the hated aspect of key ambivalent figures (the mother, the law, the devil and death) and therefore helped to allow for the staging of Oedipal wishes and the resolution of Oedipal ambivalence. Taking the "punch" out of Punch removes all of the tension and the messiness of ambivalence. Perhaps, that's not the way to do it.

To conclude

We began this chapter by looking at the outbreak of zombies on film, arguing that the zombie figure is a representation of some of the tensions of ambivalence we experience in our relationships with our semblables but which are unstageable by other cultural and/or subjective means. We find further support for this idea in our observation that in times of poor tolerance of expression of difference and intersubjective conflict, zombie film production spikes. The first of these spikes takes place in the 1970s, the second in the late 1980s; we see such spikes as radically interpretable, as saying something via film which is otherwise somehow unsayable at these times. This would point to something taking place in the preceding years which has a powerful effect upon film-makers and audiences so as to lead to a massive increase in film production. In the decade before the first of these spikes, racial tensions between black and white America were at a peak (allegorized in Georgio Romero's *Land of the Living Dead* from 1968), and during the 1980s some 25 million people died of the AIDs virus, the so-called "gay plague," unleashing a moral panic of epic proportions involving a huge increase in paranoia, fear and prejudice around gay men in particular. It is hardly insignificant that zombie films, especially from the 1980s, feature the motif of infection as the near-dominant cause of zombification.

We are encouraged to believe in the idea that 21st-century Western subjects are largely contented under neoliberalism and its attendant ideologies and practices, having swallowed wholesale the injunction to "love thy neighbor as thyself." However, we believe that neoliberalism is injected (perhaps infected, in keeping with the spread of zombiism) with all the *jouissance* psychoanalysis associates with the super-ego and its imperatives. At present, the only site where the speaking being can risk speaking outside of the terms of the politically correct in its attempted neutering of difference is the psychoanalyst's consulting room. Psychoanalysis has long attested to the symptom formation associated with the guilt – and anxiety – around wishing or dreaming that a horrid fate will befall a "loved one." What psychoanalysis observes is that today's subject, supposed to be free of hatred and hostility for his loved ones, his friends, and his neighbors, finds no place for the discharge of his/her less favorable affects and ideas concerning the people in his/her life, since increasingly, and especially under neoliberalism, it is his/her "love" for the neighbor, even while it is the very same one with whom he/she must compete under capitalism, which is nurtured and, in fact, demanded.

Notes

1. Neoliberalism refers to the political economy that underlies the functioning of capitalist societies in our times. Neoliberalist ideology revolves around the idea that reregulation of capital liberates its potential for growth and the natural tendency of the market towards equilibrium. Neoliberalism posits that competition is the defining characteristic of the social bond, and it defines individuals as consumers whose freedoms are best actualized by buying and selling. Within the neoliberalist worldview, attempts to limit competition are conceptualized as restrictions on human freedom, and taxes and regulations should be strictly limited. Neoliberalist ideology depicts inequality as the consequence of fitting rewards for those who work hard and/or generate wealth for others in the social fabric. Efforts to reduce inequality are correspondingly cast as morally reprehensible. The deregulated market, in neoliberalist ideology, enables everyone to get their fair share of the pie.
2. In *Encore*, Lacan coined the neologism "hainamoration," or "hateloving," in place of ambivalence to highlight the point where love reverses into hatred, where the semblable is transformed into something unbearable (1975, pp. 90, 91, 100).
3. *Zombies Ate My Neighbors* is a run and gun video game developed by LucasArts and originally published by Konami for the Super NES and Sega Mega Drive/Genesis consoles in 1993.
4. Available at: www.rawstory.com/2014/02/noam-chomsky-zombies-are-the-new-indians-and-slaves-in-white-americas-collective-nightmare/
5. Available at: www.versobooks.com/blogs/736-slavoj-Žižek-at-occupy-wall-street-we-are-not-dreamers-we-are-the-awakening-from-a-dream-which-is-turning-into-a-nightmare

References

Assef, J. (2013, November). The zombie epidemic: a hypermodern version of the apocalypse. *LC Express*, 2(7).

Bernays, J. (1970). *Grundzuge der Verlorenen Abhandlung des Aristoteles uber Wirkung der Tragodie*. Sect. IV. (1857). Translated by J. I. Porter as *Outlines of Aristotle's Lost Works on the Effects of Tragedy*. (1970). In J. Billings and M. Leonard M. (eds.). (2015). *Tragedy and the Idea of Modernity*. Oxford: Oxford University Press. pp. 315–329.

Billings, J. and Leonard, M. (2015). (eds.). *Tragedy and the Idea of Modernity*. Oxford: Oxford University Press.

Bishop, K. W. (2010). *American Zombie Gothic: The Rise and Fall (and Rise) of the Walking Dead in Popular Culture*. Jefferson, NC: McFarland & Company.

Clifford, S. and King, A. (2006). *England in Particular: A Celebration of the Commonplace, the Local, the Vernacular and the Distinctive*. London: Hodder & Stoughton.

Danner, M. (2009). *Stripping Bare the Body: Politics, Violence, War*. New York: Nation Books.

——. (2010, January 21). To heal Haiti, look to history, not nature. *New York Times*.

Davis, W. (1988). *Passage of Darkness: The Ethnobiology of the Haitian Zombie*. Chapel Hill, NC: University of North Carolina Press.

Ferguson, F. (2007). Oedipus: ritual and play. In H. Bloom (ed.), *Sophocles' Oedipus Rex*. New York: Chelsea House.

Freud, S. (1913). *Totem and Taboo. The Standard Edition of the Complete Psychological Works of Sigmund Freud (S.E.)* XIII. London: Hogarth Press. pp. 1–164.

——. (1930). *Civilization and Its Discontents. (S.E.)* XXI. London: Hogarth Press. pp. 59–148.

Grigg, R. (2007). Semblant, phallus, and object in Lacan's teaching. *Umbr(a): A Journal of the Unconscious*, 1 (Semblance): 131–138.

Jackson, L. (2016). Greater than logos? Kinaesthetic empathy and the chorus in Plato's laws. In M. Johncock and E. Sanders (eds.), *Persuasion and Emotion in Classical Antiquity*. Wiesbaden: Steiner Verlag. pp. 147–161.

Kahan, D. and Braman, D. (2003). More statistics, less persuasion: A cultural theory of gun-risk perceptions. *University of Pennsylvania Law Review*, 151(4): 1291–1327.

King, S. (1981). *Danse Macabre*. New York: Everest House.

Kohut, A. (2015). Despite lower crime rates support for gun rights increases. *Fact Tank Pew Research Center*, April 17.

Lacan, J. (1975). *On Feminine Sexuality, The Limits of Love and Knowledge, 1972–1973. Encore: The Seminar of Jacques Lacan Book XX*. Edited by J.-A. Miller. Translated by B. Fink. New York and London: W. W. Norton.

——. (1990). *Television: A Challenge to the Psychoanalytic Establishment*. Edited by J. Copjec. Translated by D. Hollier, R. Krauss, and A. Michelson. New York and London: W. W. Norton.

——. (1992). Miller, J.-A. (ed.). *The Ethics of Psychoanalysis, 1959–1960. The Seminar of Jacques Lacan Book VII*. Translated by D. Porter. London: Routledge.

Laurent, E. (2014). Racism 2.0. *Lacanian Quotidien*, 371, January 26.

Leech, R. (1985). *The Punch and Judy Show: History, Tradition, and Meaning*. London: Batsford Academic and Educational.

Moon, H.-J. (2014). *The Post-Apocalyptic Turn: A Study of Contemporary Apocalyptic and Post-Apocalyptic Narrative*. Ph.D. thesis, University of Wisconsin-Milwaukee, December. Unpublished.

Ozog, C. A. (2013). *Fear Rises from the Dead: A Sociological Analysis of Contemporary Zombie Films as Mirrors of Social Fears*. MA thesis, University of Regina, Saskatchewan, January. Unpublished.

Paul 5:15 In *New American Standard Bible*, Galatians, 5:15.

Phillips, A. (2015). *Unforbidden Pleasures*. London: Penguin Random House.

Poole, W. S. (2011). *Monsters in America: Our Historical Obsession with the Hideous and the Haunting*. Waco, TX: Baylor University Press.

Rasmussen, R. L. (1998). *Children of the Night: The Six Archetypal Characters of Classic Horror Films*. Jefferson, NC: McFarland & Company.

Reeve, M. J. (2005). *Contemporary Punch and Judy in Performance: An Ethnography of Traditional British Glove Puppet Theatre*. Ph.D. thesis, Royal Holloway College, University of London, London. Unpublished.

Rodriguez McRobbins, L. (2013, February 4). Are Punch and Judy shows finally outdated? *Smithsonian Newsletter*.

Russell, J. (2005). *Book of the Dead: The Complete History of Zombie Cinema*. Godalming, Surrey: FAB Press.

Saunders, R. A. (2012). Undead spaces: fear, globalisation, and the popular geopolitics of zombiism. *Geopolitics*, 17: 80–104.

Stewart, G. (2013). *The Zombie in American Culture*. MA Eng. Lit. University of Waterloo, ON, Canada. Unpublished.

Thompson, K. M. (2005). *Apocalyptic Dread: American Film at the Turn of the Millennium*. Albany, NY: State University of New York Press.

Thompson, J. F. (2015). The rise of the zombie in popular culture. In A. L. Thompson and A. Thompson (eds.), *But if a Zombie Apocalypse Did Occur: Essays on Medical, Military, Governmental, Ethical, Economic, and Other Implications*. Jefferson, NC: McFarland & Company. pp. 11–25.

Wolcott, J. (2014). Collective American scream. *Vanity Fair*, January.

Žižek, S. (2005). Neighbors and other monsters: a plea for ethical violence. In S. Žižek, E. L. Santner, and K. Reinhard (eds.), *The Neighbor: Three Inquiries in Political Theology*. Chicago: University of Chicago Press. pp. 134–190.

——. (2008). *Violence*. London: Profile Books.

——. (2016). *Against the Double Blackmail. Refugees, Terror and Other Troubles with the Neighbours*. London: Allen Lane.

13
SUSAN STERN: *SHAM*

Geneviève Morel

In her memoir, Susan Stern muses: "I will grow old ungracefully, longing for the release of death and hating its insistent approach, and never really know peace" (Stern, 1975).[1] Few things are as troubling as the mass departure of the young people from our societies, sometimes mere teenagers, to fight a merciless war against our Western democracies, by targeting their inhabitants, the so-called *kuffars* (unbelievers), be they Muslims, Christians, Jews or atheists. Having first emerged some years ago, this phenomenon has escalated since the declaration by the Islamic State (*Daesh*), on June 29, 2014, of a "caliphate" on the territories previously controlled by Iraq and Syria. Indoctrinated by the IS online ideologists, the "jihadi" fighters submit themselves to a perverted and cruel religious doctrine, which leads to mass murder and martyrdom. From one day to the next, they deny their families and their loved ones, as well as their country, which they now hate with a passion. How and why does this happen?

Despite the many sociological, psychological and journalistic studies devoted to these questions, we are still missing a proper "clinic of terrorism" – i.e. genuine case studies. I use the somewhat controversial term "terrorism" to denote either the fact of committing violent acts against the democratic society one is living in, in order to destroy it from the inside, or because of today's "global terrorism," leaving to fight in the jihadi combat zones, especially in Syria or Iraq.

Some political scientists reject case studies, because they rightly argue that there is no "typical profile" of a terrorist. Psychoanalysis does not believe in such "typical profiles," either – instead, it focuses on individual cases, which are always singular. However, it considers that studying a single case can, in fact, be instructive or even paradigmatic, as it gives us a glimpse of something more universal. Examining the trajectory of just one of these young people can help us shed light on some of the causes of terrorism, especially the terrorism of today.

A psychoanalyst relies on the words of those he or she listens to and I have had the opportunity to speak, in a forensic or medical context, with a number of jihadists returning from Syria – those who in France have been called "*les revenants*."[2] I then decided to read other testimonies, of terrorists from different historical periods and countries. It is worth pointing out that the practice of writing one's memoirs, which has become quite rare today, was very common throughout both the 19th and 20th centuries. In France, prison directors and psychiatrists used to encourage European anarchists to write down their memories and explain their motivations, all the way to the gallows; they expected to learn from these texts something valuable for both the present and the future. For example, we have the memoirs of Émile Henry, the author of the first large-scale terrorist attack, who detonated a bomb in a busy neighborhood in Paris, as well as other anarchists. This practice survived until the second half of the 20th century and throughout the student revolts, which in many countries led to the formation of new extremist movements. A number of activists, who had gone underground for having committed acts of terrorism – especially in Germany, Italy, France and sometimes the United States – also spent their long years in prison writing their autobiographies.

As Lacan pointed out, Freud was very comfortable with autobiographic texts such as Schreber's *Memoirs*, based on which he formulated a number of crucial lessons on psychosis. Akin to the practice of free-associating in a psychoanalytic session, the author of an autobiography offers us certain thoughts, the true significance of which he sometimes ignores and which help illuminate his life and destiny. Deciphering these writings falls under the rubric of what Freud called "applied psychoanalysis."

Of course, we cannot put the late 19th-century anarchists, 20th-century revolutionaries and today's jihadists all in one bag. The context has changed and so has the style of writing. With the rise of individualism and the literary genre of *autofiction*, the memoirs of the young revolutionaries of the late 20th century focus much more on their personal motivations and intimate life than those of their anarchist predecessors. Some are of no use to us, because they are too infiltrated by ideology, which seems to efface any grasp of subjectivity; this problem has also been observed by those who care for the imprisoned candidates for martyrdom. We could also object that autobiographies are necessarily permeated by fiction, as the contemporary label of autofiction suggests. However, this does not impede our research; in any case, as Lacan argued, truth has the structure of fiction.[3] The fictional parts of these memoirs can, in fact, indicate to us something about what cannot be stated directly.

Reading and deciphering these older texts can therefore tell us much about the present time; in fact, we find some of the characteristics that we might otherwise consider quite recent. For example, the phenomenon of the "born-again" converts, who leave everything overnight to blindly devote themselves to Islam; who commit acts of terrorism in their own country or leave to fight with the IS in Syria. The anarchist Luigi Lucheni, who assassinated the Austrian Empress Sissi in Geneva at the beginning of 20th century, had "accidentally" converted to anarchism, as he himself put it, only months before his crime.

Moreover, he decided to commit a regicide – *any* regicide – just a few days before killing Sissi, also nearly by accident. Before his conversion, he had been a dutiful army soldier, appreciative of the order and discipline imposed by the military – a far cry from the anarchist doctrine. As we will see, Susan Stern of the Weathermen, a revolutionary group formed in the United States in the 1960s, whose case I discuss below, also experienced such abrupt "conversion." There are other phenomena that we can find among different extremists across space and time: youth; the importance of "fatal" couples and brotherhoods; the tendency to follow a romantic partner among women; the fierce idealism; previous dislocation; indoctrination as a reaction to the existential void; the importance of an intimate event, which then serves as a point of attraction to an ideology, and so on.

The differential importance of religion in jihadism should also be put in a historical perspective: the late 19th-century psychiatrist Dr. Regis, who had long conversations in the prison with both Lucheni and Sante Caserio (the assassin of the French president, Sadi Carnot), believed that the religious assassinations of the past, where a king was killed in the name of the assassin's faith, stemmed from the same "morbid essence"[4] as the atheist anarchists he was listening to. In his view, their dreams, visions and discourse resembled each other in every respect.[5]

The importance of ideals

In trying to understand what happens to some of these young people today, the memoirs of Susan Stern are highly instructive. They show us the crucial importance of the ideals (the ideal ego and the ego-ideal) and of the super-ego in youth extremism. They also make it clear that what the young woman is trying to find in the extremist ideology is a solution to a severe and perhaps psychotic existential divide; she is looking for an ideal image, an identity that could bring together her drives and her political ideals. She is split between her violent and sexual drives, frowned upon by her comrades, and her feminine ideal. Her example also reveals that ideology is not invincible, that the individual who submits to it must actively accept it and that it can be resisted. Lastly, her book helps us examine the urgent question of what it is that such people are looking for in extremist violence: do they wish to die in order to kill, as Robert Pape suggests,[6] or kill in order to die – i.e. is this an indirect suicide?

I was drawn to Stern's autobiography for a number of reasons, including its historical interest, because it was penned early on, soon after Stern had become involved in revolutionary politics – contrary to other Weathermen who wrote and published many years later. It therefore has the authenticity of a "contemporary" testimony and is free of all "political speak." As we shall see, Susan was also partially resistant to the group's ideology, even though she admired its leaders, especially women. She also insists, including it in the title of her book, on her female specificity, which, as I will show, is at the heart of her personal and neurotic problematic. This is particularly interesting, given that the Weatherman organization shared its historical moment with the birth of the feminist movements of the

1960s. It was permeated, including its name, by the 1960s pop-culture – much more so than in Europe, given that the latter originated in the United States. And Susan is, to my mind, much more emblematic of this than other actors of her time.

Weatherman (1969–1976): pop terrorism

As you may remember, the Weatherman was a revolutionary group borrowing its name from a Bob Dylan song: "You don't need the weatherman to know which way the wind blows."[7] The group made the song the title of its founding manifesto, written in June 1969 during a Students for a Democratic Society (SDS) convention. The ironic allusion to the imminence of revolution enabled Bernardine Dohrn, a former law student and the charismatic leader of a radical fraction of the SDS, the Revolutionary Youth Movement (RYM), to attract a bunch of SDS activists, the Weathermen. Nourished by the student revolt against the Vietnam War and racism, the SDS, sometimes called the New Left, was at the time 100,000 members strong.

Today, its history has been somewhat forgotten. In the beginning, SDS was founded in 1960 as the student section of the League for Industrial Democracy (LID), a liberal organization with anti-communist leanings typical of the Cold War. The SDS founders summarized their political positions in the *Port Huron Statement*, written in 1962 by Tom Hayden, the future California state senator. The statement supported the Civil Rights Movement for racial equality and condemned nuclear proliferation, but not the communists, which led to its split from the LID, which remained anti-communist. The communists, who created a group inside the SDS called the Progressive Labour Party (PL), took part in the April 1965 March Against the Vietnam War on Washington, which brought together 15,000–20,000 students. After the march, the number of SDS members skyrocketed, reaching 100,000 in 1969. Following the Marxist–Maoist doctrine, the PL saw the organization of the working class as its most important task; the aim of the Weathermen's June 1969 manifesto was to isolate the PL, which was trying to take control of the SDS.

One of the burning issues faced by the SDS was the question of racism. The Black Panther movement, founded in 1966 to fight for civil rights, only included black activists. It advocated the seizure of power by the oppressed peoples around the world. Under the impetus of Malcolm X, it demanded that whites fight against their own racism; this created a split in the SDS and contributed to the hardening of its discourse. Some of its members began to read Régis Debray (*Revolution in the Revolution*) and think about the potential application, in the United States, of his *foco* theory, which argued that small paramilitary groups could overthrow the capitalist system from the inside. Frantz Fanon (*The Wretched of the Earth*, 1961) and Wilhelm Reich (*Mass Psychology of Fascism*, 1930–1933) were also among their key influences. The SDS journal *New Left Notes* (*NLN*) advocated overthrowing the state and abolishing private property. The 1968 assassination of Martin Luther King triggered a wave of riots throughout the country. A number of universities, including Columbia, were occupied, posing a serious challenge to the pacifism of many students.

This was also the beginning of the women's liberation movement, supported by *NLN* articles such as *Sex and Caste* by Casey Hayden and Mary King (1966) and *The Look Is You*[8] by Bernardine Dohrn and Naomi Jaffe (1968). The year 1967 saw the formation of the first women-only groups, such as WITCH or the Redstockings.

The PL remained opposed to all deviations from classical Marxism, especially the antiracist and feminist struggles, which it saw as secondary to the class struggle. It therefore considered the Black Panther Party as reactionary, while the Weathermen wanted to learn from it. Contrary to the PL, the authors of the Weatherman manifesto called for armed struggle, echoing the global anticolonial fight. The liberation of the African-American community, considered as an internal colony of the United States, was part of this. Hence the idea of an alliance with the Black Panthers and the North Vietnam fighters. This armed struggle was to be supported not only by working-class youth, but more largely by the white American youth affected by the "contradictions of decaying imperialism." The group's name was a wink addressed to the counter-culture of this youth, which was just beginning to invent new ways of living (communes, drug taking, group sex, non-monogamy and so on).

On June 20, 1969 in Chicago, about a hundred SDS activists joined Bernardine Dohrn in founding the Weatherman. During this student "coup," she declared: "We are the SDS," thus endorsing the scission and the rapid dispersion of the members of the SDS, which never again recovered. The leaders of the new avant-garde included Bill Ayers from Chicago, Marc Rudd from New Jersey and Jeff Jones from California, all students from middle-class or wealthy backgrounds.

On March 6, 1970, on the 11th Street in Greenwich Village, New York, there was an explosion at the Townhouse, a building owned by James Wilkerson, a rich publicist whose daughter Cathy had borrowed the house to use it as a bomb-making lab with her comrades. However, one of the bombs exploded too soon, killing the young pyro-technicians working in the basement: Cathy's lover Terry Robbins and two of his friends, Teddy Gold and Diana Oughton. Cathy Wilkerson and another activist, Kathy Boudin, who were upstairs in the house, survived and managed to escape the FBI.

This is to show just how much things had accelerated in less than nine months, between the SDS split of June 1969 and the March 1970 explosion. In November 1969, the Weathermen called for three days of anti-war protest in Chicago, under the slogan "Bring the War Home!" This demonstration, the so-called "Days of Rage," became incredibly violent, with many attacks on the police and a great number of arrests. However, few students had responded to the Weathermen's appeal, showing the true collapse of the SDS.

The Black Panthers were constantly hunted by the FBI. A young activist, Fred Hampton, was killed in his bed. In late December 1969 in Flint, Michigan, the Weatherman responded by declaring a "war" against the state, thus managing to scare away other, more frightened students. The decision to go underground in order to take up armed struggle was made official via the apocalyptic speech delivered by Dohrn, in which she went as far as to defend the murder of Sharon Tate by the Manson cult, adopting the "fork salute" of four fingers held up in the air as the Weatherman rallying sign (she later claimed her speech was meant to be ironic, but it seems that nobody at the time understood this). Before the explosion at the Townhouse in March 1970, bombs had already been planted in several cities, but miraculously no one had been killed. Policemen were an explicit target ("Off the pigs!"), together with the military, who were seen as complicit in the Vietnam War.

Although the Townhouse explosion plunged the group into a state of profound mourning, it also impelled them further towards clandestinity, as they were now pursued by the FBI. Weatherman thus became Weather Underground Organization (WUO). Its new targets were symbolic and the police was alerted each time to avoid victims. Bernardine Dohrn announced the new strategy of "armed propaganda"[9] via a tape recorded at a secret location. To show that the group was serious about its "Declaration of A State of War," a New York police station was bombed less than two weeks later.[10] During the 1971–1972 period, the FBI counted more than 1,800 domestic bombings: not all of these were WUO's responsibility, because there were many other terrorist groups at the time.[11]

The majority of WUO's underground leaders gave themselves up to the FBI after 1976: the Vietnam War had ended, they had aged and had children, and, above all, they knew that the majority of the charges against them would be dropped due to procedural errors. In fact, the charges collected by the FBI's COINTELPRO programme, launched by J. Edgar Hoover against domestic political movements, were pronounced illegal in 1976. Indeed, few of the Weathermen members spent time in prison, except for those who pursued their struggle in other terrorist groups and faced charges of killing policemen during the Brink's armed robbery in 1981; this was the case of Kathy Boudin, who had escaped the Townhouse explosion, and her husband David Gilbert.

Some of the WUO leaders such as Bernardine Dohrn's husband Bill Ayers became the icons of the New American Left and published their memoirs years later; however, at times, these texts seem somewhat sugar-coated.

Epiphanies and chasms

Susan Stern published her personal journal of a Weatherwoman in 1976, a year before she died from an overdose at the age of 33. Her memoir is rarely mentioned among the books of the New Left and the Weathermen.[12] It tells the story of a tragic drifting, a fragile person who was drawn, in the name of a political ideology, into a violent movement that eventually destroyed her. Incarcerated after the violent events of 1970–1971, Stern spent her days in prison writing a detailed account of the previous years, first as a member of the SDS and later the Weatherman, spanning the period of 1966–1972 and published a year before her death.

She speaks about herself candidly; her story is written in chronological order like a logbook, fresh like a snapshot. As a regular member of the movement, she is not trying to justify the political strategy over which she had no say. Because she never reached the highest echelons of the group's hierarchy, she offers us, without any clichés, a glimpse of its life quite different from that of its leaders – Cathy Wilkerson, Bill Ayers, Marc Rudd or others – who wrote their memoirs sometimes decades after the events.[13]

Together with her then husband, Robby Stern, Susan became a member of the SDS in August 1967; she was 24 years old. The couple's relationship had been floundering and they were looking for a fresh start. After having both studied at Syracuse and Susan's teaching in a ghetto school, they left the East Coast in 1966 and moved to Seattle; Robby enrolled in a law school and Susan began a degree in social work. She was hoping, though she did not have much faith in the project, to save their marriage and escape a "drab, miserable existence." She felt inferior to her gifted husband and resented the fact that in student meetings she was generally known simply as "Robby Stern's wife."

It is Robby who offers her the first joint: in a kind of exaggerated premonition, she thinks that smoking marijuana will lead to insanity and death. On the same day, she kicks Robby out, but keeps the weed. Separated from Robby and feeling very depressed, she meets a group of hippies at a demonstration. She writes: "For the first time in my life, I felt I belonged somewhere."[14] This verdict marks a fleeting joy of having found a place. However, she quickly falls back into her depression. In fact, the entire diary oscillates between moments of losing and finding herself; each time, she has the sense of having been reborn as a new person, yet these moments grow increasingly rarer.

Her encounter with the budding women's liberation movement inspires such enthusiasm in her that she starts a feminist group in Seattle as part of the SDS. In the group, she learns to speak and be listened to by other women. She adopts a new style: she changes her glasses, wears bright red lipstick and a mini-skirt. "I developed my Style. Zip, zap, I was a new Susan Stern. . . ."[15] The alternation accelerates: each brief moment of euphoria leads to a deep feeling of loss, followed by the emergence of destructive fantasies and visions. Below are two typical examples.

One: after successfully graduating from her Master's programme in Seattle, Susan finds a well-paid job as a go-go dancer in San Francisco. She is happy, but immediately becomes obsessed by a morbid fantasy. She imagines reading the newspaper headlines: a girl like her (from New Jersey) is found dead, strangled in her topless dancer costume.

Two: at the large SDS demonstration in August 1968, during the Democratic Convention in Chicago, Susan feels "part of a great whole."[16] Feeling vindictive, she is "ready to riot": "I wanted to kill." When she is injured during the demonstration, she has terrible, quasi-hallucinatory visions, like epiphanies: she sees the dead body of Malcolm X, the lynchings of black Americans, Vietnamese babies covered with napalm.

> I thought about Auschwitz, and mountains of corpses piled high in the deep pits dug by German Nazis. I closed my eyes tightly, but tears oozed from under my lids and rolled off my face. A new feeling was struggling to be born in me. It had no name, but it made me want to reach beyond myself to others who were suffering. I felt real, as if suddenly I had found out something true about myself [. . .]. Now I would fight.

On both occasions, she describes her body as a "corpse." In the second vision, she enters a state of universal communion with all the victims of genocides and Nazism. However, it is paradoxically precisely this identification, this communion with the dead, that bring, her out of her depression, provoking feelings of elation and sustaining her desire to keep fighting.

My super-ego nickname

When the SDS splits in June 1969, Susan follows the Weatherman. She feels galvanized by the charismatic Bernardine Dohrn, although she misses the "big family" of the SDS and the feeling of belonging it gave her. She asks herself whether the split is a "suicide," but concludes that:

> listening to Bernardine, I felt that I had finally connected with my own personal destiny; that I had a place, a function in life. That place was with the Weathermen, that function was to fight for the revolution to the best of my ability [. . .] Weatherman. I fell in love with a concept. [. . .] I ceased to think of Susan Stern as a woman; I saw myself as a revolutionary tool. [. . .] my family, my past all faded into dreary insignificance. For the first time in my life that I could remember, I was happy.[17]

In her descriptions, we always find the same conjunction of a happy *rebirth* – which is reaffirmed each time, as if it was the first time – and a correlative *loss* of the ego and its possessions, where even her feminine identity becomes untenable.

In late 1969, during a demonstration into which she throws herself with abandon, Susan suffers a severe concussion and needs to be hospitalized. Her singular style is not appreciated by the Weatherman leaders, despite her efforts at self-criticism to obey their iron discipline. She then gives herself a derisory nickname – Susan Stern *Sham*.[18] In her self-baptism, the self-derisory sobriquet materializes her super-ego's agreement with the leaders' critique.

The Freudian super-ego is a paradoxical concept: its power is fueled by the guilt generated not just by actions, but also by unconscious wishes.[19] In addition, the misfortunes suffered by the ego and its renunciations are considered as faults and provoke further punishment by the super-ego, which can then lead to actions against the law. The super-ego gradually becomes more and more ferocious; it expands, fueled by the death drive and destructiveness unbound from the erotic libido. When Susan is disparaged and punished during the criticism sessions, not only does she accept her punishment, but her super-ego amplifies it further – hence the adoption of this intimate nickname, a sign of her downfall. Still, she remains with the Weathermen, even though she has been quarantined. The leaders eventually exclude her completely when they decide, in December 1969 in Flint, to go underground. Susan hopes to re-enter the organization, but instead falls into a deep depression.

In spite of this, the hope for a new rebirth never leaves her. In March 1970, she reads about the Townhouse explosion, just after her divorce from Robby has been finalized. She decides to go underground with another small revolutionary group, the Seattle Liberation Front, but eventually changes her mind. In a moment of despair, wishing to end with it all, she collects her old letters and notebooks, her poems and photos from her youth, and throws everything away, together with the beautiful clothes her father had given her:

> Soon there would be no more Susan Stern. She would be dead, and the person she had been would have another face, another color hair, another name, another past. She would invent it, build it, engineer it to be exactly what she wanted it to be, what she had never been. [. . .] A past of fiction, a life of science fiction. Susan Stern Sham would end finally, finally she would end.[20]

To sacrifice everything: her possessions, her ego, her image, her female identity and finally even her name and nickname. And, *in fine*, her life. The perpetual repetition of these losses seems to be the necessary precondition for the glimmering and vain hope of a mythical reconstruction, not just of the present, but also of her past.

Dream-o-lution[21]

But it is not yet 1970. Previously, Susan is passionately devoted to her revolutionary beliefs, but also remains lucid, as if she was not completely taken in by the Weatherman propaganda – a contradiction that contrasts with the blind obedience of her fellow activists.

Constantly concerned about her femininity, she is particularly interested in the new feminist movements such as National Organization of Women (NOW). She has a hard time tolerating the dominance of certain male leaders, who abuse the so-called *sleeping rule* (everyone must sleep with everyone) to bend their female comrades to their will. Although she feels attracted to the "great" leader Bill Ayers, she refuses to go to bed with him, because he behaves too much like a "superstar."[22] Still, she feels obliged to sleep with a certain "JJ," simply because he saved her from the cops. She becomes more resistant to the "Crush Monogamy" slogan when she finds a regular lover, Garrity, with whom she also does drugs. Unfortunately, Garrity is not part of Weatherman.

Some leaders are dismissive of her – for example, Marc Rudd. The loudmouths always win: "There was no way to escape the fact that I was white, female, from a wealthy family, Jewish, had been married, was well educated, had been a ghetto school-teacher, etc. The obvious reaction to Rudd's contempt for me never crossed my mind; he was from a similar background."[23] She also struggles with the criticism of another leader, Kathy Boudin, who sidelines her, even though Susan does her best to perform various menial tasks in order to be accepted: "She frightened me to death. [. . .] Kathy seemed above sexual need, beyond the petty and childish fantasies I still secreted about falling in love and being loved."[24] At the same time, she is not blind to the barely disguised *jouissance* that these admirers of Mao's Red Guards derive from the criticism sessions they impose on others.

Susan dreams of the big day to come: "In my dreams of revolution was a world where class and race had vanished, and only peace, love and happiness remained."[25] Yet her dream is crushed by the collapse of the SDS. There were 500,000 of them in the United States, a big community open to everyone, but all that ended with the "Big Split. Not immediately. But inevitably. [. . .] Pig paranoia became a plague [. . .]." Even though she has followed Bernardine Dohrn with great enthusiasm, Susan looks towards the future without any illusions. Also, she has no say over it. "I wandered away from the Seattle group with a growing sense of alarm and isolation. Somehow the die had been cast, the split was on, but did I personally want it? It had nothing to do with me, really. I was just a plebeian; the leadership had made the decision, and now it was a fact. How was I related to this fact?"

At the same time, she is not ready to obey blindly. After one last criticism session, when she is reproached for her eccentricity, her drug habits and above all the shocking contradiction between her revolutionary feminist ideals and having earned her living as a go-go dancer, the Weathermen Seattle collective decides to exclude her from the local leadership. When she is invited to come back shortly afterwards, she refuses. She wants to stay in the group, but keep her freedom: "I was a Weatherman cheerleader. I was a religious zealot. I was a crazy fool in love with the notion of revolution without any idea of its concept."[26] She believes that the Weathermen destroy instead of constructing; she does not want to submit. She concludes: "As much as I loved Weatherman, I loved my individuality more." She keeps her high heels and her miniskirt; she refuses to adhere to the sleeping rule. She accepts her contradictions. She even consents to the criticism sessions enforced by the leadership, because she believes that transformation can be achieved at the cost of losing oneself. However, does she not already indulge in this type of process on her own? Despite her fascination with the leaders she admires, she knows very well they are mistaken and refuses to join in what she considers abuse. Susan Stern is perhaps a sham, but she is not just a pawn.

Suicides on repeat

Susan's ex-husband Robby decided never to follow the Weathermen. He would mock them, asking her ironically if they were planning to kill all white Americans. He admonishes her right from the start: "You didn't start seeing things that way when you became a revolutionary. You have always done these numbers behind suicide." In his view, the Weathermen simply provided a social and political pretext to Susan's pre-existing suicidal tendencies.[27]

Indeed, Susan speaks about a series of suicide attempts during her childhood. When she was 3 years old, her mother, "beautiful and childlike," left the family home for another man, whom she loved "more than her children." Susan and her younger brother Roger were thus separated from their mother at a very young age. After a brutal legal battle that lasted six years, the custody of the children was given to the father, a rich businessman who adored and spoiled his daughter. It is evident that Susan perceived the mother's leaving as an abandonment and that this was constantly emphasized to her by her father.

In this dramatic context, Susan first attempted suicide at the age of 13. Her father slaps her, because he thinks that he saw her in a car with her mother. This is not true and the girl, who is suffering greatly from the separation, answers that she has not seen her mother for months. The father does not believe her; in response, she swallows an overdose of pills.[28] Susan speaks about this first attempt when she describes another, in late 1969, after the Weatherman convention and the "declaration of a state of war" in Flint, a time when she felt "untouchable." During one of the endless criticism sessions she is asked, in order to free herself from her bourgeois upbringing, to sleep with a couple she likes. She cannot comply. In addition, the sudden decision of the Weathermen to go underground in order to take up arms leaves her speechless: she refuses to leave the world in this way. Overnight, she is then kicked out of her small local Weathermen community. "And then I got the idea. Suicide! [. . .]. And here I was at the age of 27, still as emotionally unequipped to deal with myself as I was at 13." Feeling transformed into a "worm, disgusting, foul," she swallows a lethal dose of Seconal, a dangerous barbiturate. By pure chance, her lover Garrity finds her unconscious and saves her. It is no coincidence that her autobiography makes a connection between these two suicide attempts: the first has to do with being let down by the mother, which is confirmed by the father. The second is a repetition of this abandonment by the Weatherman leadership, which for her functions as the law.

This is the beginning of Susan's desperate and suicidal drifting from one group to another. Looking for an alternative to the Weatherman, she joins another group, Sundance, named after the film *Butch Cassidy and the Sundance Kid*, the very same that inspired the desire to "go out in a blaze of glory" in Teddy Robbins, the bomb-maker of Townhouse. The members of Sundance practice a kind of "festival of *jouissance*." Occasionally, Susan also spends time with another revolutionary group, the SLF, where she sleeps with any man available and takes a lot of drugs.

She falls into a spiral of violence. With her comrades, she prepares "The Day After" in Chicago, a demonstration to protest the trial against a group of demonstrators, the "Chicago Seven," seen as unjust. Susan hopes that she will get herself killed:

> I was obsessed with death and dying. I began to think about bombing the police station again, making sure I perished in the explosion. I fantasized about shootouts with a dozen pigs, killing some of them, and finally getting killed myself. I daydreamed of setting an ROTC building on fire, and burning to death in the blaze. My death had to count for something. I couldn't just die anymore; I had to die with meaning. My life couldn't be wasted by a wasted death. In those days before TDA, I was consumed with murder and suicide and violence.[29]

However, after this post-demonstration, the Sundance leaders exclude her from their group as well, describing her behavior as "kamikaze." Susan herself is still excited by the sound of the broken windows. When she hears about the Townhouse explosion, she experiences a wave of self-hatred at the idea of still being alive: "I hated my flesh, my breath, my nose, my feet. I despised the tenacity with which I clung to it. My thoughts swung even more morbidly. If one could not live meaningfully, one at least could die meaningfully. That much control one had over one's life." In other words, she downright envies the three Townhouse victims.

As her husband said, Susan Stern had suicidal aspirations since childhood; these then morphed into her revolutionary ideas and quickly became accentuated. As we have seen, she even dreams about being killed with a gun in her hand. During the Days of Rage she carries a revolver and learns how to make Molotov cocktails. After her trial in 1970, she leaves for the mountains with a chemist, to learn how to handle dynamite. She speaks about her visions of blowing up the IBM and Boeing factories: "We hated America. [. . .]. Our hearts were in the hills, with our bombs; our hearts were underground, with the Weathermen."[30] Susan would like to give her own death the same revolutionary meaning as the one she ascribes to the Townhouse victims. At the same time, this idea and practice of violence animate and galvanize her, keeping her alive like a regular dose of speed: the planned death is thus suspended each time, but for how long?

The Weatherwoman: how to heal the fatal flaw?

Stern is able to formulate the division that is gnawing at her: "My sexual desires came from a different part of me than my revolutionary ideals [. . .]." Faced with this split between her sexual drives and her ideals, she feels terribly alone.[31] During the summer of 1970, she tries to put this division into action, on one hand, through rampant bodily practice: "sex, dope and violence!" is her slogan; on the other hand, by devoting the rest of her time to the secret implementation of her revolutionary project – i.e., making reliable bombs. However, this solution is not quite satisfying.

Susan tries to overcome the division she could not assume in different ways. First, she tries to the conceal it by the "ideal image" of the female revolutionary, Bernardine Dohrn, whom she has admired since their first meeting in the SDS:

"The way she spoke and moved; such control, such self-assurance, such elegance. She immediately became a symbol of what I hoped to become. At the same time, I felt helplessly inadequate in the face of all that splendor."[32]

The desire to serve a political cause cannot be separated from a certain conformism vis-à-vis the avant-garde, an attitude that can be traced back to childhood. Already as infants, we can sense our parents' expectations. These eventually form an "ego-ideal," a reference point that we use to transform our ego into an "ideal ego," the image that will satisfy the parents. The coupling between the ego-ideal and the ideal ego[33] functions throughout life: in the family, at school, in the army, at university, at work, in the couple, and so on. Each time, the subject tries to identify with the ideal ego defined by the elder or the boss, by the loved, envied or admired person who embodies the ego-ideal. And each time, the success of this identification coincides with the feelings of exaltation experienced as being freed from the "ordinary yokes" of the past.

Bernardine is therefore the ideal ego before whom Susan inevitably feels miserable. During the Days of Rage they are arrested together. Even after being thrown into the police van, Bernardine retains her charm:

> She looked like a fashion model. Short black leather jacket, nice slacks, neat purple blouse, the boots – everything just so. [. . .] I just plainly stared at her, unable to fathom the source of her charisma. She possessed a splendor all of her own. Like a queen, her nobility set her apart from other women.[34]

Later, Susan listens, transfixed, to the diva's first underground communiqué: "It was like a voice from heaven, from the future, a voice that no American law could silence." She is also impressed by other women, such as the beautiful Cathy Wilkerson, who takes the time to listen to her life story – as opposed to her mother, to whom Susan could never explain anything, given how much the mother was preoccupied with her own problems. Or, in a negative way, Kathy Boudin, who galvanizes her during a demonstration, but later turns very critical towards her and whose militant rigidity "frightens [Susan] to death."[35] The feminine ideal thus becomes the sarcastic voice of the super-ego.

The other way of stitching together the two sides of her division would be, of course, to try to embody the ideal image of the leader herself. Yet Susan cannot succeed at this; her division deepens and inexorably tears her apart. When she tries to be a "serious revolutionary," she imagines herself covered in blood on the streets of Chicago. During the Days of Rage, which are broadcast on TV in "gory Technicolor," she thinks: "The whole world is watching [me]."[36] However, this image of a fighter again gives way to the sexy image of the go-go dancer, who is rejected by other Weatherwomen, because she stands for the objectified woman, at odds with their revolutionary ideals. As we already know, this eventually leads to Susan's exclusion, because her behavior is excessive on both fronts – on the side of the struggle and the side of femininity.

Nevertheless, she does have one opportunity to mend this inner breach, by bringing her image as a woman and a Weatherman fighter together: during the Seattle Seven hearing, a trial against a group of anti-war activists, where she is one of the defendants. She feels very important, having become *the* female voice of the revolution. She is the "lone woman defendant" and identified as such "a hundred times" by the press: "Suddenly I was someone. [. . .]. And finally, no one but me to undertake the tremendous responsibility of being the female voice which would be carried to other women across the country."[37] Since all the top Weatherwomen have gone underground after the Townhouse explosion, "it was my voice which would be heard at rallies, mine in classrooms, mine in newspaper interviews, radio talk shows, and over the news. [. . .] since I had been singled out by the government, other women wanted to know what I knew." Susan has found a mission. During this period, she becomes friends with Annie Anderson, a devoted activist who supports her during the ensuing difficult months, in the course of which she suffers from various physical issues: STDs, an unwished-for (and long denied) pregnancy, an incurable cold, the effects of her drug use, etc.

Thanks to this new (imposed) mission, Susan manages to take on the ideal image of the revolutionary woman. She is preoccupied with what to wear to the hearings; she alternates, "between my long black skirt and black hat and knitting like Madame DeFarge [the *tricoteuse* of the French Revolution in Dickens's *A Tale of Two Cities*], and my miniskirt for a little shock therapy." In this outfit, she manages to plead and also deliver a political speech, despite the judge's attempts at preventing her from doing so.

However, the relief brought by the unifying image of the female revolutionary is short-lived. Susan quickly falls back into depression and drugs – evidence that she is not a paranoiac, because no mission seems to sustain her for very long.

She then decides – this is her third attempt at healing her split – to write her memoirs, starting in the prison where she has been sentenced for six months. She describes her mental state to her friend Anne:

> Still, I am unhappy in my role as a revolutionary, because it is not enough for me; I want to stand out in the history I am trying to make. My existence will have meaning only if lots of others know about it. Call it fame, immortality, call it what you will, until I have it, I will always be unhappy. I guess that's the saddest thing about me, my *fatal flaw*.[38]

However, writing is not enough to stabilize her, although she manages to publish her memoir in 1975. A year later, after another romantic disappointment, she dies from an overdose in what seems to be a barely concealed suicide. Her political adventure was born from the breakdown of her marriage to Robby; she kills herself after her latest romantic failure. The story comes full circle, especially if we think of her abandonment, as a young child, by her mother, her suicidal attempt at 13, linked to the pain of this separation, and what she was looking for later among women – namely, an ideal, but also someone who listens, which her own mother was never able to do (we have seen that she mentions this when speaking about Cathy Wilkerson). She also writes to Anne: "Love, I almost hate the word. I have always been an abysmal failure at it. I have always thought if I could find love I would not crave fame so, but it seems I lose on both scores."

Today like yesterday?

Susan Stern's activist and terrorist trajectory seems paradigmatic of the youthful appetence for the excitement of extremism and the swift passage to the act. In her case, we can indeed speak of terrorism, despite her modest discretion regarding her acts, probably due to the risks of legal persecution: when her book was published in 1975, the Weathermen were still active underground and carrying out bomb attacks. Although she does not say very much about this, Susan nevertheless mentions that she continues to make explosives and that she carries guns during demonstrations – presumably to use them.

Her political engagement was serious, even though she always trailed behind those she depended on (her husband and later Bernardine Dohrn) and never devoted herself to studying revolutionary texts (she says that she barely skimmed through the Weatherman manifesto). However, she never agreed to submit herself to the rules that bothered her, such as "Smash Monogamy," nor did she conform to stereotyped gender behavior. This ambivalence shows us that action can be prompted by an image rather than a theorized political engagement and even though one does not quite agree with one's leaders. Today's terrorists are often described as radical individuals completely at one with their ideology; yet in reality they can be ambivalent; they might hesitate for a long time, before suddenly carrying out their mad acts. Susan is a good illustration of this type of behavior.

Finally, it is the ideal image of the female revolutionary that magnetizes her, that is her "divine inspiration" – the woman she meets and whom she would like to become.[39] For a brief moment, this image heals the painful split between her drives and her ideals, by condensing the violence that inhabits her with her ideal. The image of the revolutionary woman makes her a "passionate idealist," a term coined in 1913 by the French psychiatrist Maurice Dide.[40]

Her revolutionary involvement seems to resemble that of other students of her generation: protesting the Vietnam War and racism. However, it is based on a singular constellation.

During one demonstration, as she is getting ready to fight against the "Nazi state," ready to kill and be killed, Susan has a fleeting thought of her father. The source of her torment is her suspicion that this rich Jewish capitalist had learned nothing "from the massacre of six million Jewish human beings in Germany."[41] Susan thinks of her father as a racist who hates people of color and other religions. We remember her vision of a pile of bodies, in the sinister communion with all of the victims of genocides and of Nazism, which led her to experience herself as a corpse. From now on, Susan is situated alongside these massacred victims, while her father, who in a sense has foreclosed his Jewish origins, is located on the other side – of the white men she is fighting against, the killers, the pigs. Susan also blames her father's cruelty for her suicide attempt at 13. However, at the same time, she remains her father's daughter, claiming her white bourgeois and Jewish origins. She brings all of these identities together and does not deny either of them: on one hand, she identifies as a victim of massacre; on the other, she is the killer of white men, of pigs like her father. This further strengthens her sense of guilt.

Because of the latter, she obeys the punitive super-ego that pushes her to go kamikaze *in a version that is above all suicidal*: rather than killing, she wants to be killed, but only as long as she finds a glorious death. Her super-ego, precociously engendered by the void of her mother's abandonment, which the father did not manage to make up for, is feminine and lawless. It takes on the seductive traits of the great Weatherwomen, in fact capricious superwomen like Bernardine Dohrn or Kathy Boudin. Susan's constant preoccupation with her image and reputation resembles the concerns of other terrorists such as Terry Robbins, whose glorious end – "dying in a blaze of glory," as in the final scene of *Butch Cassidy and the Sundance Kid* – she envies.

Notes

1. Stern, S. (1975). *With the Weathermen. The Personal Journal of a Revolutionary Woman.* New Brunswick, NJ: Rutgers University Press, p. 363.
2. After the bestselling book by the French journalist David Thomson.
3. See Lacan, J. (2001). Litturaterre. *Autres écrits.* Paris: Seuil, pp. 12, 13.
4. Of course we do not believe in the existence of any such "morbid essence" – it is a term of 19th-century psychiatry.
5. Régis, E. (1890). *Les régicides dans l'histoire et dans le présent: étude médico-psychologique.* Paris: A. Maloine.
6. Pape, R. A. (2005). *Dying to Win, The Strategic Logic of Suicide Terrorism.* New York: Random House. According to Pape, even in 2001 the kamikaze fighters continue to commit altruistic suicides in Durkheim's sense – they sacrifice themselves for the benefit of others and a political cause.
7. Dylan, B. (1965). "Subterranean Homesick Blues."
8. Dohrn, B. and Jaffe, N. (1968). *The Look Is You: Toward a Strategy for Radical Women.* Women's Liberation.
9. Burroughs, B. (2015). *Days of Rage, America's Radical Underground, the FBI, and the Forgotten Age of Revolutionary Violence.* New York: Penguin Books, p. 122. For the Weatherman's *Declaration of A State of War* see: www.youtube.com/watch?v=jbpTvkp Zluk
10. Berger, D. (2010). *Weather Underground. Une histoire explosive du plus célèbre groupe radical américain.* Paris: L'échappée, pp. 212–214.
11. Burroughs, B. (2015). Meet the Weather Underground's Bomb Guru. *Vanity Fair,* March 29, 2015.
12. She is not at all mentioned in, for example, the books by Dan Berger, Cathy Wilkerson or Bill Ayers, even though the latter two were her comrades.
13. Wilkerson, C. P. (2007). *Flying Close to the Sun. My Life and Time as a Weatherman,* New York: Seven Stories Press; Ayers, B. (2001). *Fugitive Days. A Memoir.* New York: Penguin Books; Rudd, M. (2009). *My Life with SDS and the Weathermen Underground.* New York: William Morrow.

14. Susan Stern, op. cit., pp. 11 and 14.
15. Ibid., pp. 21–22.
16. Ibid., pp. 20, 34, 36.
17. Ibid., p. 72.
18. Ibid., pp. 191 and 208.
19. Freud, S. (1930). *Civilization and Its Discontents. S.E.* XXI. London: Hogarth Press, pp. 57–146.
20. Ibid., p. 249.
21. *Rêve-lution* in the original.
22. Ibid., p. 76.
23. Ibid., pp. 42, 43.
24. Ibid., p. 59.
25. Ibid., pp. 66, 62, 68, 69.
26. Ibid., pp. 96 and 123.
27. Ibid., p. 98.
28. Ibid., pp. 230, 231.
29. Ibid., pp. 236, 237, later 241 and 244. Emphasis mine.
30. Ibid., p. 271.
31. Ibid., p. 252.
32. Ibid., p. 47.
33. Freud, S. (1914). *On Narcissism. S.E.* XIV. London: Hogarth Press, pp. 67–102.
34. Ibid., pp. 150, 151 and 268.
35. Ibid., p. 59.
36. Ibid., pp. 136, 137.
37. Ibid., pp. 260, 264.
38. Ibid., p. 363. Emphasis mine.
39. Ibid., p. 112.
40. Dide, M. (2006). *Les idéalistes passionnés* (1913). Paris: Frison Roche.
41. Stern S., op. cit., p. 135.

References

Ayers, B. (2001). *Fugitive Days: A Memoir.* New York: Penguin Books.

Berger, D. (2010). *Weather Underground: Une histoire explosive du plus célèbre groupe radical américain.* Paris: L'échappée. pp. 212–214.

Burroughs, B. (2015). *Days of Rage, America's Radical Underground, the FBI, and the Forgotten Age of Revolutionary Violence.* New York: Penguin Books. p. 122.

—— (2015, March 29). Meet the weather underground's bomb guru. *Vanity Fair.*

Dide, M. (1913/2006). *Les idéalistes passionnés.* Paris: Frison Roche.

Dohrn, B. and Jaffe, N. (1968). *The Look Is You: Toward a Strategy for Radical Women.* Women's Liberation.

Freud, S. (1914). *On Narcissism. The Standard Edition of the Complete Psychological Works of Sigmund Freud (S.E.)* XIV. London: Hogarth Press. pp. 67–102.

—— (1930). *Civilization and Its Discontents. (S.E.)* XXI. London: Hogarth Press. pp. 57–146.

Lacan, J. (2001). Litturaterre. *Autres écrits.* Paris: Seuil. pp. 12, 13.

Pape, R. A. (2005). *Dying to Win, The Strategic Logic of Suicide Terrorism.* New York: Random House.

Régis, E. (1890). *Les régicides dans l'histoire et dans le présent: étude médico-psychologique.* Paris: A. Maloine.

Rudd, M. (2009). *My Life with SDS and the Weathermen Underground.* New York: William Morrow.

Stern, S. (1975). *With the Weathermen: The Personal Journal of a Revolutionary Woman*. New Brunswick, NJ: Rutgers University Press. p. 363.

Wilkerson, C. P. (2007). *Flying Close to the Sun: My Life and Time as a Weatherman*. New York: Seven Stories Press.

14

BREAKING THE SPELL OF THE SLAVE REVOLT IN MORALITY

From the subreption of identity-in-difference to the repetition of the paraconsistent

Alireza Taheri

Aligning Freud with Kant, Copjec reads the primal murder as a "noumenal" event, one that cannot be an object of experience. She introduces the notion of "subreption" to denote the operation through which "a supersensible idea" is "falsely represented as if it were a possible object of experience" (Copjec, 1996). The subreption of the primal murder corresponds to representing this event as something one may experience, a deed not yet realized. This has "the effect of both exonerating us of the murder and making us guilty of its nonaccomplishment" (ibid.: xxii). The subject thus falls prey to the super-ego that punishes "severely every failure of will to realize itself" (ibid.: xxii). Obstacles to the realization of this crime are vilified as impediments to a delusional notion of freedom. Expanding on Copjec's use of Kant, I redefine Kantian subreption as the failure to recognize the (noumenal) identity of pairs, which, within (phenomenal) experience, are felt as opposed.[1] I show how apparent contraries such as truth and lie, religiosity and atheism as well as Good and Evil (to name a few) only appear opposed through subreption. If, as François Balmès (2007) argued, for every statement by Lacan one can find the opposite claim, this I argue, because apparently opposed pairs conceal affinities that the common understanding cannot fathom. Symbolic castration represents an unreachable ideal point where the subject is reconciled with the identity of opposites and is not captive to the illusion of their phenomenal contradiction. Beyond the emotional difficulties (the pain of mourning loss), symbolic castration represents a challenge to ordinary cognition: how can two things that seem stringently opposed constitute a deeper identity? Throughout my argument I show how the failure to reckon with identities-in-difference relegates the subject to deeper contradictions that define central aspects of our contemporary predicament.

In a passage from *Less than Nothing* concerned with no less than "the negativity which founds the symbolic order itself" (Žižek, 2012, p. 860), Žižek argues that "primordial repression" is not the repression of something into the unconscious but a repression constitutive of the unconscious. Insofar as it involves the expulsion of the real into the symbolic, this "*Ausstossung*" appears as a process diametrically opposed to "*Verwerfung*" entailing the foreclosure of a signifier into the real. Žižek paradoxically argues, however, that *Ausstossung* and *Verwerfung* occur simultaneously in the founding gesture of the symbolic order. The expulsion of the real into the symbolic cannot occur without the exclusion of a signifier from the symbolic order thus constituted: "The price the symbolic has to pay in order to delimit itself from the Real is its own being-truncated" (ibid., p. 863). For the symbolic order to have consistency it must, paradoxically, be deprived of something. The failure to recognize this identity-in-difference (the symbolic order's lack is also its support) involves subreption, the most radical form of which is the specific foreclosure involved in psychosis.[2] The failure to fathom the constitutive paradox of the symbolic order relegates the subject to the central contradiction of psychosis – namely, a "full" symbolic order devoid of lack which is, paradoxically, all the more depleted. The emergence of the subject also requires the simultaneous operation of *Ausstossung/Verwerfung*. If *Ausstossung* corresponds to the expulsion of the real through the intervention of speech and the articulation of desire, *Verwerfung* points to the ineradicable alienation this entails: "desire is *inarticulable* precisely insofar as it is articulated in a signifying chain" (Žižek, 1996, p. 6). The subject is decentred in the Other ("desire is the desire of the Other") and, Žižek reminds us, this Other is also decentered. The act of speech through which the subject asserts herself is paradoxically tantamount to alienation. As Žižek notes, Agamben shows that "'desubjectivization' ('alienation') and subjectivization are thus the two sides of the same coin: it is the very 'desubjectivization' of a living being, its subordination to a *dispositif*, which subjectivizes it" (Žižek, 2012, p. 984). The psychotic subject, neither "desubjectified" nor alienated, is all the less "subjectified."[3]

Ausstossung/Verwerfung requires elevating the father's particular enunciation to the status of universal Law. The difficulty of the paternal function lies in that it involves the gesture by which a particular poses as universality. We here encounter the discrepancy between the real and symbolic father. The latter places himself beneath the Law that he proclaims. In terms of Lacan's (2001) formulae of sexual difference, the symbolic father says: "all are subject to castration" (for all x, Φ x). By contrast, the *real* father, as agent of castration, cannot enforce this Law all too "democratically." He imposes castration while excluding himself from it as he sexually enjoys his wife. The father now says: "there is one that is not subject to castration" ($\exists$x, not Φ x). The point from which the incest taboo is pronounced is a point of its transgression.[4] As Žižek (2012) says, echoing Brecht, "what is a crime against the Law in comparison to the crime that is the Law"? To institute the All of castration, we must accept the paternal exception. Insofar as he assumes the place of exception, despite being the voice of the universal, his position cannot be duplicated;

there cannot be two exceptions. As Allouch (2004) says, the father is "non-specularisable" insofar as he is the One and only exception to the All of castration. The symbolic father of universal castration is noumenally equivalent to the perverse super-egoic father, though the two are experienced as radically contrasting. This disparity provides yet another index of the difficulty of fathoming castration.

Interestingly, Žižek defines radical Evil as a particular's pretence to pose as the universal. Evil is thus not "particularity as such but its false, 'perverted' unity with the universal." In Evil, the universal is debased "to a mere means of my self-assertion" (Žižek, 1996, p. 15). If the paternal function requires that a particular father represent the universal incest taboo, then the subject's acceptance of this universal interdiction requires a paradoxical acceptance of a paternal radical Evil. In proclaiming the Law – and yet exempting himself from its jurisdiction – the real father becomes a figure of radical Evil; the father's *voice*, in all its *jouissance* and particularity, poses as the agent of universal castration. If the father is "a sacred reality, more spiritual than any other" (Lacan, 1981, p. 244, my translation) and if Evil is "incomparably more spiritual, remote from sensual *Genuß*, than is the Good" (Žižek's, 1996, p. 18), then is the father not the embodiment of a radical "spiritual Evil" insofar as he represents, as Žižek's Schelling would say, the "false unity of Ground and Existence"? Before cynically equating paternity and Evil, we must remember that the father's intervention will be *seen* as Evil only insofar as the subject is not duped by the paternal word. The real father may facilitate this duping if he assumes his position with irony. If, like the proverbial king, the father really thinks he is a father, then we would be really dealing with radical Evil – namely, a particular man debasing the universal to his own self-assertion. The unduped subject sees Evil in the field of the Other and she will respond with Evil, her only means of protest. Instead of a subject assuming alienation in a symbolic order that is itself decentered, we have two figures of radical Evil in a struggle of pure prestige. First, we have the Evil of the symbolic order imposing its *particular* symbols in a false pretence to universality. Second, we have the Evil of a subject refusing to acknowledge reliance on these symbols in a posturing of autonomy. A subject who does not relinquish his defiance against the paternal Law will transform the latter, in fantasy or delusion, into a monstrous Thing. As Hegel says, "Evil resides in the gaze itself which perceives the object as Evil" (Žižek, 1998).

If the subject is duped, then she will achieve the symbolic murder of the primal father. The movement towards the universality of Law occurs through this radical "crime." We must avoid idyllic readings that emphasize the primordial "yes" or "*Bejahung*" to the father without underscoring the crime at the base of peaceful co-existence. Where the constitution of the subject and the symbolic order are concerned, Evil has primacy over the Good. Radical Evil, or the death drive, makes possible the advent of the subject; it is, Žižek argues, the act of "deciding one's eternal character" or, in Lacan's words, "the unsoundable decision of being" (Lacan, 2006, p. 177). By accepting a paternal Law that contradicts its content through its very enunciation, the subject paradoxically achieves a symbolic murder of the father. The latter is a radical ethical *act* through which emancipation occurs.

If symbolic castration is operative, neither the father's Word nor the subject's act will be seen as Evil. Responsibility for this act will thus be possible.

In psychosis, the subject is not duped by the Other and, for this very reason, remains passive to the Other. Being duped by the Other and subverting it belong together. This paradox is captured by the tension between two stories of enormous import for psychoanalysis. The first is the myth of the murder of the primal father and the second is the biblical story of Abraham and Isaac.[5] The former narrates the tale of the necessity of sacrificing the primal father who stands in the place of the Other of *jouissance*; the primal figure of obscene enjoyment must be abolished for the sake of social co-existence. The latter, by contrast, relates the need to sacrifice the son. Rather than choose between these alternatives, we must posit their noumenal identity such that the primal murder may *only* take place as the subject assumes his symbolic death. Insofar as the vocation of man is that of a *son*, we must all first die by a suicidal act of faith through which symbolic castration occurs – this is Isaac submitting himself to Abraham's knife. Only then, paradoxically, will we have successfully killed our fathers and opened for ourselves a margin of freedom.

Coetzee's *Disgrace* tells the story of a white South African woman raped by two black men. Her decision to keep the child attests to the courage of admitting the unconscious. Her maternal joy must be contrasted to the cowardly sadness of rejecting the unconscious and shunning responsibility for the moral weight it casts on the subject. She realizes that true freedom requires accepting that freedom and enslavement are only opposed from the limited perspective of subreption. Hegel's master–slave dialectic provides a brilliant evocation of the identity-in-difference of slavery and mastery: the master's freedom leads to impasse while the slave's labor opens the way for possible freedom. Perhaps with the advent of capitalism and the decline of feudalism, the identity-in-difference of the master and slave was subject to increased subreption as the capitalist–laborer relation of domination took its place. This subreption may arguably account for the countless contradictions of the capitalist mode of production outlined by Marx.

The ethical act, Žižek (1996) argues, has the same form as radical Evil insofar as neither is motivated by egotism. Žižek thus posits the identity of Good and Evil with the claim that "Evil is 'Good in becoming'" (Žižek, 2003, p. 88). In similar vein, for Badiou, Evil is not the outcome of ignorance but the consequence of an "over-fidelity" to a truth:

> As can be seen with scientism, or with totalitarianism, there is always a desire for the omnipotence of the True. There lies the root of Evil. Evil is the will to name at any price. Usually it is said that Evil is lies, ignorance, or deadly stupidity. The condition of Evil is much rather the process of a truth.
>
> (Badiou, 2003, pp. 66–67)

Evil is the Good that has lost its sense of measure. The challenge of symbolic castration is here felt with all its ethical weight as the subject is beckoned to recognize the formal equality of the most heinous Evils and the loftiest Goods. The failure to recognize this formal identity relegates us to the mediocrity of compromise formations in the realm of ethics.

The symbolic murder of the father is essential for the advent of the symbolic order and the subject; it is the radical *Ausstossung* through which the subject gains respite from the monstrous Thing. This primordial *Ausstossung* manifests as a decision to speak and articulate desire. The subject abandons the silence of *infancy* and joins the community of speakers. However, insofar as *Verwerfung* must accompany every *Ausstossung*, the subject's speech will be tainted with a stain of falsehood; she is forced into a minimal lying gesture as the truth may be spoken only through the medium of untruth. If symbolic castration occurs, this minimal lie at the basis of all enunciation will not be seen as Evil. For the psychotic subject, the lie is impossible and concomitantly the dimension of truth is devoid of efficiency. The lie accompanying truth as its shadow plagues the psychotic with melancholic guilt when observed in himself and paranoid rage when witnessed in the signs of the Other. What he cannot fathom is the fictional structure of truth, or, in our terms, the noumenal identity of truth and lies.

Symbolic castration is a matter of faith. It is thus no surprise that religiosity is so vastly targeted in psychosis. However, atheism is also abolished insofar as true atheism and religiosity belong together. The noumenal identity of faith and atheism lies in the fact that both involve symbolic castration; religion and atheism without castration correspond, respectively, to fanaticism and scientistic/dogmatic materialism. The escalation of religious fanaticism and new religiosities as well as the rise of vulgar materialism (e.g. Dawkins's (1989) claim that intelligent life emerges only when an organism discovers evolution) represent, according to Žižek, two sides of the same coin. We could say that both miss the identity of atheism and religiosity. The atheist's rage against religion (e.g. Hitchens's (2007) puerile "God is not great") and the fundamentalist's fury at the heathen's faithlessness are manifestations of "the suicidal aggression of narcissism" (Lacan, 2006, p. 174) where the subject does not see that it is "precisely the *kakon* of his own being that [he/she] tries to get at in the object that he strikes" (ibid., p. 175). Lacan rejects Nietzsche's infamous "God is dead" as "a shelter against the threat of castration" (Lacan, 1977, p. 27) as well as Dostoevsky's idea that the inexistence of God would lead to everything being permitted (Lacan, 2007). We have Nietzsche the atheist and Dostoevsky the theist, but what is missing is their identity-in-difference.[6] Lacan's "God is unconscious" (1977, p. 59) may provide the formula for this atheism as religiosity.

A similar paradox lies at the level of the Law. Modern legal thought promotes an objective conception of the Law (Goodrich and Carlson, 1998, p. 1), thereby obfuscating the tie connecting Law and desire. By contrast, psychoanalysis reveals the "Law's unconscious, its 'other scene'," (ibid., 1998, p. 3). For Legendre, desire itself is at work in the Law as the subject's "love of the censor" (ibid., 1998, p. 9). The desire inherent to the Law splits it from within, thereby making it inconsistent. However, psychoanalysis reveals the paradox according to which the force of the Law, its power, is tied to its frailty. When Lacan claims that the "symbolic father is, strictly speaking, unthinkable" (Lacan, 1994, p. 210, my translation) he means that no father can hold his symbolic mandate without delegitimizing it with a taint of personal *jouissance*. The wager, however, is that without this blemish, the father's authority falls. To have causal efficiency, the Law must be tainted by failure. Common understanding cannot grasp this paradox and thus denies the inconsistencies of Law in the hope of establishing an "objective" Law. Philosophical/psychoanalytic reason tells us that an "objective" Law is deprived of force. Moreover, such an "impotent" Law leads to more oppressive forms of subjugation. This is the university discourse with its principle contradiction according to which an "objective" Law without force is all the more tyrannical. This leads to a further contradiction at the level of the subject: the "free" and "equal" subject of liberal democracy is more than ever constrained by what Schütz calls a "theo-technological power, which is incontrovertible [and] speechless" (Schütz, 1998, p. 206).

Drawing on Agamben (1998), Santner (2011) explores the contradiction by which the subject of university discourse is at once "sovereign" and "bare life." Like the medieval king, this subject has two bodies – one made sublime through symbolic investiture and the other made abject by the threat of social upheaval. With the decline of paternal authority, children are today's sovereigns. The child who is the object of maternal *jouissance* has two bodies wavering from the privilege of having the mother's unique attention to being haunted by a possible castration which, foreclosed from the symbolic, may return in the real, thereby confirming the body's abject destitution. In Althusserian terms, we witness a decline of the ideological apparatus of the family. Formerly, the family was the principle ideological apparatus (with the Church and education apparatuses also having important roles) responsible for assuring symbolic castration. Today, we see the child's direct encounter with the ideological apparatus of psychiatry and, what is worse, the repressive police apparatus. The danger is that the child's confrontation with such apparatuses is far more terrifying than former negotiations with parents. Moreover, punishment in the hands of the police can no longer claim the expiatory power it had when delivered by the hands of parents.

Insofar as the family ideological apparatus is the home of symbolic castration minimally guaranteeing subjectivity, the negative designation of "ideology" requires further elucidation. The family represents the beginnings of the encounter with the values of society. A tremendous process of internalization takes place through which social substance marks itself on the flesh. The Name-of-the-Father allows for some respite from this subjugation, enabling the child to work through trauma in an on-going neurotic questioning. Repressive apparatuses, Althusser explains, leave little room for flexibility (Althusser, 2014, p. 248), while ideology has a "double character"; it is a *recognition* in the form of *misrecognition* or an *allusion* in the form of an *illusion* (ibid., p. 259). Ideological apparatuses are founded upon fictions (ibid., p. 252), while repressive apparatuses appeal to force in brute reality. As fiction is the condition of truth, the loss of the family threatens the space of working through where truth may emerge in the interstice of fiction, where recognition may occur in the site of misrecognition and where an allusion to a subject is made in the midst of illusion.

Though psychiatry is situated in the domain of ideology, it harbors a more distant relation to subjective truth than family. Here, fiction, illusion and misrecognition do not readily pave the way to truth, allusion and recognition. Some ideological apparatuses are arguably more conducive to truth and subjectivity. Perhaps the older feudal apparatus of the Church, like the family, also provided a space commensurate with truth and subjectivity. One should not undervalue the potential for subjective truth concealed within Christianity's mystifications. Indeed, family and Church have much in common. First, both appeal to paternal authority. As Kojève explains (2014), the authority of the father was theoretically elaborated by scholastic philosophy and theology. Second, the Christian religion is arguably founded on a "family romance" (the virgin mother, the immaculate conception) and, conversely, biblical stories offer allegories for the dramas of family life (the story of Abraham and Isaac delivers an unparalleled metaphor of symbolic castration). Third, faith plays a prominent role in both; the religious man must take a leap to enter the community of believers, as the "good son" must give his "yes" to the father to partake in the privileges of family.

The constricted spaces of psychiatry and disciplinary power are not abodes for myths through which truth emerges. A subject relegated to the apparatuses of police and psychiatric power finds reconfirmed in the Other his paranoid defiance against society. Family enables the ever-renewed construction of fantasies – ideologies commensurate with the growth of subjectivity. It functions through a central paradox hinging on the identity-in-difference between submitting to the Law and finding refuge from it: *one must say "yes" to paternal authority in order to thereby gain some freedom from the family*. Psychotic children who refuse this affirmation are more tightly bound to the family, seldom leaving home – so much for the "nomadic" schizophrenic. Likewise, the paradox of faith is that atheism is possible only for those who do not relinquish Christianity – something Žižek has argued in his effort to reveal the materialist potential of Christianity. Those who cannot grasp this remain bound to the contradiction of naive atheism where vulgar materialism enslaves the subject more stringently to the Other. The liberating identity-in-difference through which adherence to an ideology affords respite from that ideology is less likely to operate in medical ideology where the subject faces the contradiction of increased subjugation with every effort towards freedom – the more passionately one claims sanity, the more the medical straitjacket is enforced. The scientistic space of psychiatry leaves little space for truth and the thriving of subjectivity. This is truer for the repressive apparatuses where Agamben's (2009) sinister idea of subjugation without subject is a looming threat.

The current dissipation of the boundaries separating public and private has to do with the failure to fathom the identity-in-difference between externality and interiority – namely, the idea that intimacy/interiority require sociality. Numerous ways in which Lacan theorizes this identity-in-difference could be isolated: 1) the notion of "extimacy" (a portmanteau word combining "external" and "intimate"); 2) the topology of the Moebius; 3) the claim according to which the "unconscious is politics" (Lacan, session of November 11, 1966). Simply put, deprived of public life, the subject also loses access to interiority. The failure to fathom this identity-in-difference has arguably led to the contradictions involving the encroachment of private obscenity into public space and vice versa (e.g. social media) as well as the contradictions related to sexual life attested to in the growth of sex without love/intimacy (the increase of pornography and dating sites) and in the rise of love without sexuality (sexless marriages). As a result of this conflation (public and private), the "mirror stage" has taken on a peculiar form as the "clinical gaze" of psychiatry and the disciplinary measures of the Law have replaced the mother's holding gaze and the father's loving voice. For some, the psychiatric label and the criminal record are the last vestiges of identity for bodies otherwise reduced to bare life. Althusser's notion of interpellation arguably represents a reformulation of the mirror stage in light of the late modern decline of family. In the past, institutions liminal to the public and the private, such as the school or the Church, provided further spaces where castration could be symbolically instantiated. Today, the repressive apparatus is a veritable emergence of castration in the real resulting in Foucaultian "carceral archipelagos" (Foucault, 1975) such as Goffman's "fugitive communities" testifying to "the massive expansion of criminal justice intervention into the lives of poor Black families" (Goffman, 2014, p. 249), where the "dirty" subject – the colloquial inner-city name for what Agamben (1998) would call "sacred life" – is forced into exemption from whole sectors of public life.

Such are the consequences of the university discourse's struggle with the contingency of power. For Žižek, the way out of this contingency is through its redoubling in the figure of the monarch standing at the helm of the social edifice. Without the repetition of the contingency of Law in the figure of the monarch we err into the university discourse. Within the family a similar problem occurs when the redoubling of contingency fails – namely, when the father fails to embody Law while also standing outside it. The escape from the "caprice" of maternal Law is not achieved by grounding her power in necessity (by reading endless books on parenting, for instance) but by *repeating* this contingency in the figure of the father as family "monarch." Analogous difficulties result within the therapeutic setting when the analyst does not occupy the place of sovereign. This occurs either when the analyst maintains the position of a *subject supposed to know* or when she opts for transparency and erases any trace of difference in power. The Lacanian scansion reintroduces sovereignty in the analytic session, thereby opening the space of the treatment – without a sovereign exception there is no transference. The cure involves the realization that the analyst is not a subject of knowledge but, rather, someone more akin to the Žižekian–Hegelian "idiotic" monarch there to "dot the 'i's" – namely, to simply "return the analysand's own message in an inverted form."

For Žižek, "the exercise of authority is an 'irrational' act of contingent decision which breaks the endless chain of enumerating reasons *pro et contra*" (Žižek, 2012,

p. 430). In today's democracies, the act is stifled by the incessant speech of what Donoso Cortés christened the "discussing class" (Schmitt, 1985) – namely, the liberal bourgeoisie. The slave revolt in morality involves what Schmitt diagnosed as the ubiquitous "onslaught against the political" (ibid., p. 65) where endless parliamentary debates replace the political. If, as Badiou (2013) holds, Nietzsche is the thinker of the "archi-political," it is because he fought most stringently against the "democratic prejudice in science" (Nietzsche, 1998) that has obliterated authority and installed the reign of endless chatter. Psychoanalysis as "conflictual science" (Althusser, 1999) must also resist the slave revolt in morality; it cannot regress to dialogue. The decline of the political implies the demise of the therapeutic. The neologism "politico-therapeutic" may thus denote the common object of Marx's critique of political economy and Freud's discovery of the unconscious and help us better appreciate that the Law is at once political and intimate, political because intimate. The slave revolt in morality grounds the end of the politico-therapeutic and paves the way for the triumph of the university discourse, the antithesis of the conflictual sciences. With the decline of the politico-therapeutic, late modernity testifies to the daunting contradiction of subjugation – interpellation without subjectivity, a predicament akin to madness.

Bidet explains that, for Althusser, interpellation is a "pact" of freedom and equality (Bidet, 2014, p. xxviii). This pact has not only failed to fulfill its promise but, by dint of the contradictions of capitalism, has led to greater enslavement. The "class struggle," Bidet argues, "expressly appeals to [the interpellating discourse] as a promise which, as such, should be kept" (ibid., p. xxvii). Our late modern predicament reveals us as the dupes of a "broken promise." Taking a spin on Lacan, we could say that we are today both *duped* and *erring*. If we take the reference to *promise* as evocative of love as a symbolic *pact* (Lacan, 1988, p. 197), then we must conclude that we today, dupes of a broken promise, are the fools of unrequited love. Here the "death of God" takes an uncanny turn; his death signals our desertion and the loss of hope that our love will be reciprocated. Like the erotomanic subject, we are ecstatically in love with the absolute Other with no hope of requital other than in delusion.

Žižek (2012) argues that we live today in a world dominated by the "paraconsistent" logic that rejects the principle of non-contradiction while adhering to the principle of the excluded middle term. Among today's many contradictions, we have isolated, to here rename a few, the fact that the Law without force leads to greater tyranny and that the sovereign subject is reduced to bare life. Nietzsche has never been more of a contemporary; today, he truly weeps as we enter the reign of the slave revolt – namely, the triumph of the university discourse and its paraconsistent contradictions. Under the slavish revaluation of values, the slave is master and defeat is victory as the meek are the new bearers of the emblems of honour.[7] For Badiou (2008), change has to be sought in "classical" logic endowed with the highest potency of negation as it endorses both the principle of non-contradiction and that of the excluded middle term. However, Žižek has shown that our solution cannot consist of classical negation since, under the auspices of the paraconsistent logic, "negation gets caught up in the game" (Žižek, 2012, p. 1010). Where the slave revolt dominates, negating it will only result in its inexorable triumph. In a paraconsistent world, we must opt instead, Žižek argues, for the logic that rejects both the principle of non-contradiction and that of the excluded middle term – this is the road of the weakest negation. We may link this to Žižek's defence of monarchy – a veritable middle term that breaks the paraconsistent logic by which slave morality co-opts every defeat into a reconfirmation of its hegemony and that also rejects the principle of non-contradiction as this "monarchy" is self-annihilating such that the king is an "idiot" that "dots the 'i's'," the father a "dead" and "humiliated" figure, and, finally, the analyst but a "dummy" echoing one's message. Rather than stark negation, our paraconsistent world requires repetition. Badiou (2008) bemoans the paraconsistent where "everything is identical." Moreover, he fails to think the affirmation of repetition, something Nietzsche (1969) ardently celebrates as the "marriage ring of rings" – namely, the eternal return. If "the wound can be healed only by the spear which smote it" (Žižek, 2004), then nothing is more opportune than repeating the paraconsistent. Deleuze (1968) does not lament the state where all is the same since the repetition of the Actual is the condition of true change at the level of the Virtual. Instead of the classical negation of Law, we need to think the event in terms of paraconsistent repetition. If, as Badiou himself argues, a certain excess in the situation is "at once the guarantor of the being of presentation [. . .] and what threatens to subvert its Law" (Brassier, 2007, p. 106) and if, according to Žižek (2009), the super-egoic underside of the Law is our only prospect of emancipation, then the repetition of the paraconsistent logic – which recognizes the hidden identity between Benjamin's (2007) "mythic Lawmaking" and "divine Law-destroying" violence – is our only hope today of breaking the spell of the slave revolt in morality. Through repetition, the paraconsistent logic – heir to the Hegelian dialectic – sublates into the desired logic that rejects both aforementioned principles and thereby opens a third way beyond the endless chatter of the "discussing class" and Nietzsche's nostalgia for antique lands – two options we must rigidly discard lest we wish to keep on weeping.

I have set the common understanding against philosophical reason throughout my argument. However, it is crucial to bear in mind that this opposition too is an effect of subreption. In the noumenal domain (an ideal point we can never reach), reason and the understanding coincide. In other words, the misperception by which, say, true religiosity (e.g. Hegel's notion Christianity) and atheism are opposed harbors, though implicitly and in the form of misrecognition, the kernel of the truth regarding their identity. If truth and lies mask a secret identity, then the errors/lies of the understanding are perhaps our only means to access the truths of reason (recall that for Lacan (1977), "there is no truth that, in passing through awareness, does not lie"). Perhaps Žižek is trying to get at something similar when, positing "the identity-and-difference between Understanding and Reason" (Žižek, 2016, p. 45), he argues that "Reason is Understanding itself in its productive aspect" (ibid., p. 46). Likewise, the noumena–phenomena opposition collapses at the noumenal level as it can only perdure under the spell of subreption. But even at the phenomenal level, it collapses because here the noumenal is out of reach. One expression of the noumena–phenomena identity is found in the fact that the dream is at once the "royal road to the unconscious" (Freud, 1900) as well as the quintessential domain of the mirages of the imaginary. The subreption of this identity is responsible for the scientistic relegation of the dream to meaningless non-sense as well as its obscurantist elevation to oracle or divination. By insisting on the identity-in-difference of noumena and phenomena, we are repeating Žižek's move from epistemology to ontology – namely, the move from Kant to Hegel–Lacan. The unknowability of the world is henceforth not a consequence of human limitation but, rather, of the essentially "not-all" or incomplete–inconsistent character of the world itself: "*the limitation of phenomena is not external but internal*, in other words [. . .] the field of phenomena is *in itself* never 'all', complete, a consistent whole" (Žižek, 2012, p. 283). There is thus only a phenomenal realm and the so-called noumenal is nothing other than phenomenon's non-self-identity; or, as Žižek puts it, "there is no need for any positive transcendent domain of noumenal entities which limit phenomena from outside – phenomena with their inconsistencies, their self-limitations, are 'all there is'" (ibid., p. 283). We may apply this argument to the aforementioned contraries: religiosity's non-self-identity makes it identical to atheism, truth's non-self-identity equates it with fiction and lie, the Good's non-self-identity equates it to Evil, and so on. If "nothing, either in heaven or on earth [. . .] exhibits the abstract 'either–or' as it is maintained by the understanding" (Hegel, 1991, p. 187), then speculative reason may help uncover these identities-in-difference. Against Badiou, we must here hold that the paraconsistent does not posit a drab identity between all things. Rather, it posits the specific identity of opposites through which the said non-self-identities may be better apprehended. A genuinely paraconsistent thought will take us in the direction opposed to subreption where seeming contraries are naively set against each other.

The slave revolt in morality is the ethical, "archi-political" name of the thorough-going subreptions resulting in the contradictions plaguing the times. Subreption involves the imaginary degradation of the symbol through which, for instance, the Law appears in the perverted form of the super-ego as "deferred obedience" (Freud, p. 1913) to the father. Three such imaginary degradations corresponding to the three structures of the subject may be isolated. Neurotic psychical subreption, known as repression-denial, leads to the phenomenalization of the object *a* aimed at obfuscating the horror of castration. Eventually, castration triumphs as neurotic guilt where the subject is persecuted by this very same object *a* returning as a menacing internal voice. Perverse psychical subreption involves the erection of a fetish in the service of disavowal. Commenting on a boy whose disavowal was immediately followed by a symptomatic fear concerning his toes being touched, Freud announces the implacable triumph of castration: "in all the to and fro between disavowal and acknowledgment, it was nevertheless castration that found the clearer expression" (Freud, 1938, p. 278). Finally, psychotic psychical subreption, known as foreclosure, leads to a manifestation of castration in the real where the subject is confronted with an "unbarred" persecutory Other. In all three cases the identity-in-difference of lack and the phallic function is subrepted, thereby leading to three contradictions defining each structure. In neurosis, we have a subject who refuses "to sacrifice his castration" (assuming that the Other demands it of him (Lacan, 2006, p. 826)) but who, for that reason, remains all the more bound to his castration. In perversion, we have a desire that puts on the aura of subverting the Law while functioning as the very support of Law (Lacan, 2004, p. 176). Finally, in psychosis we have a subject sheltering herself from the Other for fear of becoming its object; what she cannot fathom is that the effort to ward herself off reifies her all the more. In all cases the identity-in-difference of castration (loss) and desire (gain) is subrepted. Some *jouissance* must be lost to access desire. When this fails, we are trapped in the daunting contradiction where castration itself becomes a source of insufferable *jouissance*. Our late modern culture of *jouissance* testifies to this; we live in the contradictory times where the gap between enjoyment and pain is hardly discernible.

The son may inherit his father's masculinity only at the cost of submitting to the father's phallic power. Without this primary feminization, masculinity will founder. Put aphoristically, *it is only the daughter in the son that will ever grow to become a man*. The subreption of the identity of masculinity–femininity has led, at the social level, to various contradictions regarding gender. On the "conservative" end, we have excessive masculinity coexisting with impotence (men's movements growing as a result of the current frustration of masculinity), while on the "liberal" end we have the discourse of transsexualism which thinks itself forward-thinking while anachronistically appealing to an essentialist "error of nature."[8] At a theoretical level, the subreption of sexual identity-in-difference leads either to 1) the impasses of essentialism where sexual difference is solidly grounded in nature or to 2) "postmodern" approaches where difference is relegated to the ruses of ideology. Regarding the latter, a central error of Butler's (1997) work is that she takes a certain contradiction regarding sexual orientation (heterosexuality as "melancholic" identification caused by the unmourned loss of the homosexual other) as constitutive of sexuality rather than as a specific outcome of the contemporary subreption of sexual identity-in-difference. Where the essentialist posits difference as incontrovertible, the postmodernist insists on identity. Both miss the specific dimension of sexual identity-in-difference upon which alone castration is sustained.

Our aim to counter subreption overlaps with that of the psychoanalytic cure – namely "to raise impotence to impossibility" (Lacan). This task requires reckoning with the challenge that the paraconsistent poses to the common understanding. It is our failure to recognize the paraconsistent logic of identity-in-difference that will leave us at the mercy of the contradictions of late modernity. If we cannot acknowledge guilt and accept symbolic castration, as Kant urges when he pleads for "an unconditional obedience of moral Law" (Copjec, 1996), we will not be freed from the defences against guilt in which Adorno (2010) rightly saw the origins of modern violence. If we cease trying to fathom the coincidence of contraries, we will find ourselves at the mercy of the ghastly contradiction which Freud (1916) so elegantly christened as "criminals out of a sense of guilt" and which Nietzsche named the "pale criminals," a humanity reduced to "a coil of wild serpents that are seldom at peace among themselves [. . .] seeking prey in the world" (Nietzsche, 1969, p. 66).

Notes

1. Following Copjec's lead, I adopt this Kantian terminology as it provides a clear framework for my argument. Later I show how my thesis concerning deeper identities perceived as differences must also be applied to the noumena–phenomena distinction, thereby absolving the Kantian structure of my argument. This theoretical move follows the transition from Kant to Hegel as theorized by Žižek; this is the move from epistemology to ontology.
2. The general foreclosure or *Verwerfung* constitutive of the symbolic order must be distinguished from the specific foreclosure of psychosis, which concerns a particular signifier, the Name-of-the-Father (see Maleval, 2000). We may relate these together by arguing that the specific foreclosure of psychosis is tantamount to the subreption of the general foreclosure constitutive of the symbolic order and subjectivity.
3. If we follow Lacan's claim that "the madman is the free man," (Lacan, 1969, p. 17, my translation) we must add that this "freedom" is identical to servitude.
4. Lacan argues that "the parent of the same sex appears to the child as both the agent of sexual interdiction and the example of its transgression" (Lacan, 2001, p. 46, my translation). Here too, however, we must be attentive to the logic of identity-in-difference lest we overlook the fact that the father's potency hinges precisely on his castration. If the father can successfully transgress the Law, he proclaims it is because he has submitted to his own father's Law. It may arguably be the case that the subreption of this identity-in-difference (castrated father = potent father) has led to the contemporary crisis of paternity marked by the contradiction of the simultaneous rise of "humiliated" fathers on one hand, and perverse seductive ones on the other, not to mention that these two opposed figures are often imagined to co-exist in the same person.
5. Serge Leclaire's tellingly entitled *A Child Is Being Killed* begins with a reference to Abraham and Isaac as a metaphor for the psychoanalytic process. The child that is "killed" is the "imaginary phallus" – namely, the object of maternal desire that forms the kernel of the ego in the mirror stage.
6. Incidentally, the failure to recognize the identity-in-difference of atheism and religiosity may explain the glaring contradictions of Dostoevsky and Nietzsche's personal lives, a pious sinner on one hand and an impious saint on the other.
7. The most comical and yet most distressing of today's contradictions is undoubtedly the fact that toddler-sized hands control the world's greatest nuclear arsenal.
8. Regarding the use of the phrase "error of nature" in transsexualist discourse, see Gherovici (2010, p. 165).

References

Adorno, T. (2010). *Guilt and Defense. On the Legacies of National Socialism in Post-War Germany*. Translated, edited and with an Introduction by J. Olick and A. Perrin. Cambridge, MA: Harvard University Press.

Agamben, G. (2009). *What Is an Apparatus? and Other Essays*. Translated by Kishik and Pedatelio. Stanford, CA: Stanford University Press.

Agamben, G. (1998). *Homo Sacer. Sovereign Power and Bare Life*. Stanford, CA: Stanford University Press.

Allouch, J. (2004). *Ombre de ton chien. Discours psychoanalytique, discours lesbien*. Paris: Epel.
Althusser, L. (1999). *Writings on Psychoanalysis: Freud and Lacan*. New York: Columbia University Press.
Althusser, L. (2014). *Initiation à la philosophie pour les non-philosophes*. Texte établi et annoté par G.M. Goshgarian. Paris: Presses Universitaires de France.
Badiou, A. (2003). Philosophy and truth. In O. Feltham and J. Clemens (eds. and trans.) *Infinite Thought. Truth and the Return to Philosophy*. London and New York: Continuum Books. pp. 58–68.
——. (2008). The three negations. *Cardozo Law Review*, 29(5): 1977–1983.
——. (2013). Le séminaire. Lacan. *L'Antiphilosophie (1994–1995)*. Paris: Textes établi par Véronique Pienau. Ouvertures. Fayard.
Balmès, F. (2007). *Dieu, le sexe et la vérité*. Toulouse: Éditions Érès.
Benjamin, W. (2007). On violence. In *Reflections: Essays, Aphorisms, Autobiographical Writings*. Edited by P. Demetz. Translated by E. Jephcott, Preface by L. Wieseltier. New York: Schocken Books.
Bidet, J. (2014). Introduction: An invitation to reread Althusser. In Althusser, *On the Reproduction of Capitalism. Ideology and Ideological State Apparatuses*. Preface by E. Balibar. Introduction by J. Bidet. Translated by G. M. Goshharian. London and New York: Verso.
Brassier, R. (2007). *Nihil Unbound. Enlightenment and Extinction*. London: Palgrave Macmillan.
Butler, J. (1997). *The Psychic Life of Power. Theories in Subjection*. Stanford, CA: Stanford University Press.
Coetzee, J. M. (1999). *Disgrace*. London: Vintage Books.
Copjec, J. (1996). Evil in the time of the finitude world. In J. Copjec (ed.), *Radical Evil*. London: Verso Books.
Dawkins, R. (1989). *The Selfish Gene*. Oxford: Oxford University Press.
Deleuze, G. (1968). *Différence et répétition. Épiméthée*. Paris: Presses universitaires de France.
Foucault, M. (1975). *Surveiller et punir. Naissance de la prison*. Paris: Gallimard.
Freud, S. (1900). *The Interpretation of Dreams. The Standard Edition of the Complete Psychological Works of Sigmund Freud (S.E.)* IV. Translated by J. Strachey. London: Hogarth Press.
——. (1913). *Totem and Taboo (S.E.)* XIII. London: Hogarth Press.
——. (1916). *Some Character-Types Met with in Psycho-Analytic Work (S.E.)* XIV. London: Hogarth Press.
——. (1938). *Splitting of the Ego in the Process of Defense (S.E.)* XXIII. London: Hogarth Press.
Gherovici, P. (2010). *Please Select Your Gender. From the Invention of Hysteria to the Democratizing of Transgenderism*. New York and London: Routledge.
Goffman, A. (2014). *On the Run: Fugitive Life in an American City*. Chicago: University of Chicago Press.
Goodrich, P. and Carlson, D. G. (1998). Introduction. In P. Goodrich and D. G. Carlson (eds.), *Law and the Postmodern Mind. Essays on Psychoanalysis and Jurisprudence*. Ann Arbor, MI: University of Michigan Press.
Hegel, G. W. F. (1991). *The Encyclopaedia Logic*. A new translation with Introduction and notes by T. F. Geraets, W. A. Suchting, and H. S. Harris. Cambridge: Hackett Publishing Company.
Hitchens, C. (2007). *God Is Not Great*. New York: Hachette Book Group.
Kojève, A. (2014). *The Notion of Authority (A Brief Presentation)*. Edited and introduced by F. Terré. Translated by H. Weslati. London and New York: Verso.

Lacan, J. (1966–1967). *The Seminar of Jacques Lacan.* Book XIV. *The Logic of Phantasy.* Translated by C. Gallagher from unedited French manuscripts.
——. (1969). *Petit discours aux psychiatres.* Conférence au cercle d'étude dirigé par H. Ey, inédit, p. 17.
——. (1977). *The Seminar of Jacques Lacan.* Book XI. *The Four Fundamental Concepts of Psychoanalysis* (1963–1964). Edited by J. Allain-Miller. Translated by A Sheridan. New York and London: W. W. Norton.
——. (1981). *Les psychoses.* Séminaire III. Text prepared by Jacques-Allain Miller. Paris: Éditions du Seuil.
——. (1994). *Le séminaire. Livre IV. La relation d'objet.* Paris: Le Seuil.
——. (2001). *Autres Écrits.* Paris: Éditions du Seuil.
——. (2004). *Le séminaire. Livre X. L'angoisse.* Paris: Le Seuil.
——. (2006). *Écrits.* Translated by B. Fink. In collaboration with H. Fink and R. Grigg. New York and London: W. W. Norton. (Page numbers refer to the French original displayed in the margin of the text.)
——. (2007). *The Seminar, Book XVII. The Other Side of Psychoanalysis,* 1969–1970. Edited by J.-A. Miller. Translated by R. Grigg. New York: W. W. Norton.
Leclaire, S. (1975). *On tue un enfant.* Paris: Éditions du Seuil.
Maleval, J.-C. (2000). *La Forclusion du nom-du-père. Le concept et sa clinique.* Paris: Éditions du Seuil.
Nietzsche, F. (1969). *Thus Spoke Zarathustra. A Book for Everyone and No One.* Translated by Hollingdale. London and New York: R. J. Penguin Books.
Nietzsche, F. (1998). *On the Genealogy of Morality.* Translated by M. Clarke and A. Swensen. Cambridge: Hackett Publishing Company.
Santner, E. (2011). *The Royal Remains: The People's Two Bodies and the Endgames of Sovereignty.* Chicago: University of Chicago Press.
Schmitt, C. (1985). *Political Theology. Four Chapters on the Concept of Sovereignty.* Translated and with an Introduction by G. Schwab. With a new Foreword by B. Strong. Chicago: University of Chicago Press.
Schütz, A. (1998). Sons of the writ, sons of wrath: Pierre Legendre's critique of rational law-giving. In P. Goodrich and D. G. Carlson (eds.), *Law and the Postmodern Mind. Essays on Psychoanalysis and Jurisprudence.* Ann Arbor, MI: University of Michigan Press.
Žižek, S. (1996). Selfhood as such is spirit: F. W. J. Schelling on the origins of evil. In J. Copjec (ed.), *Radical Evil.* London and New York: Verso.
——. (1998). For a leftist appropriation of the European legacy. *Journal of Political Ideologies,* February.
——. (2003). *The Puppet and the Dwarf.* London: MIT Press.
——. (2004). The politics of redemption. Why is Wagner worth saving? *Journal of Philosophy and Scripture,* 2(1): 18–30
——. (2009). De la démocratie à la violence divine. In *Démocratie, dans quel état?* Paris: La Fabrique.
——. (2012). *Less than Nothing: Hegel and the Shadow of Dialectical Materialism.* London: Verso.
——. (2016). *Disparities.* London: Bloomsbury Academic.

15

TERROR AND THE UNCONSCIOUS

Psychoanalysis in Argentina, 1976–1983

Patricia Gherovici

When I left Argentina having trained there as a Lacanian psychoanalyst, my friends told me to forget about psychoanalysis because in the United States, psychoanalysis had been killed. Of course, this was an exaggeration, but, as Theodor Adorno once quipped, of psychoanalysis nothing is true but exaggerations. Indeed, I was leaving behind Buenos Aires, the so-called world capital of psychoanalysis. In Argentina, psychoanalysis was extremely popular and as much of a national symbol as soccer, tango, the disappeared and the Madres de Plaza de Mayo. This chapter focuses on the astonishing popularity of psychoanalysis in Argentina in a complex political context that combines a history of state terror and dictatorships with a robust clinical practice and cultural presence of psychoanalysis. This chapter attempts to find a rationale for the wide appeal of psychoanalysis in violence-plagued Latin American locations and apply the lessons gained to other geopolitical contexts.

"Forget about Freud, Lacan and above all, psychoanalysis. Psychoanalysis is dead in the United States." First, let me give you some context for such an ominous prediction. I was leaving behind Buenos Aires, the so-called Paris of South America and also the world capital of psychoanalysis – Argentina leads the world in the shrink ratio: in Argentina, whose population is 41 million, there are 81,000 psychologists, not too far from the number of psychologists in the US – 93,000 to be precise – yet for a population eight times bigger. What is more, in Argentina to be a psychologist means one thing – to be psychoanalytically oriented.

While one does not need to go too far to see that the influence of psychoanalysis in the United States is waning, psychoanalytic practice continues to flourish around the world, particularly in Latin American locations ravaged by varied forms of violence, ranging from extreme poverty to state terror. Not only is the cultural presence of psychoanalysis in Argentina great, its adoption is wide ranging and it is never a stigma. On the contrary, people include this piece of information in their résumés, even listing with pride the name of the analyst and the number of years they have been in treatment. In Argentina, time spent on the couch at least increases your respectability – you may suffer, but you want to do something about it.

In the country of tango we are all psychologists: 85% of psychologists in Argentina are women and 75% work in clinical practice. Alejandro Dagfal (2009) studies this singular phenomenon and talks of an "invention of the psychologist" in Argentina, where the close relationship between the psychologist and psychoanalysis has led to an extraordinary expansion of the practice of the unconscious in what he calls "the Argentinean psychological exception." Most psychoanalysts have a Lacanian orientation. Dagfal has studied this phenomenon showing that Lacan is more alive in Argentina than in France. Dafgal argues that the transformation of psychoanalysis from a counter-cultural discourse into the dominant discourse was driven by the creation in 1957 of the profession of psychology at the prestigious university of Buenos Aires. Up to then the practice of psychoanalysis had been relegated to the medical domain. With the creation of the profession of psychology, very soon being a psychologist and a psychoanalyst became synonymous.

Since the late 1950s psychoanalysis has been systematically taught at university level and the career formation of psychologists has meant an academic education in psychoanalysis. Mariano Plotkin calls the position of psychoanalysis in Argentina's psychological community "hegemonic." Furthermore, being a psychoanalyst is considered better than being a psychologist. In my own personal experience, I graduated as a psychologist from the University of Buenos Aires in 1988; my studies in psychology meant five years of graduate studies in psychoanalysis – even the syllabus of courses in psychology like statistics or projective testing techniques included texts by Lacan, which at times felt like some sort of disclaimer to justify the deviation from pure psychoanalysis imposed by the demands of a program that was supposed to be in psychology.

In the city of Buenos Aires alone, we find more than 25,000 psychoanalysts. Psychoanalysis is embedded in the geography of its main city, where there is a tree-lined district affectionately nicknamed Villa Freud, a neighborhood mostly populated by analysts and analysands. Let us not assume that doing psychoanalysis is just considered to be "chic," as one would conclude looking at the crowds of neurotics, fashionably dressed and pensively lingering in Villa Freud's cafés. No. Psychoanalysis is everywhere. From seasoned politicians to hairdressers, to soap opera stars to bank tellers, everyone uses psychoanalytic terms to express themselves in everyday life. Ordinary Argentines offer psychoanalytic interpretations at the drop of a hat and can hold forth with precision on the difference between Freudian and Jungian methods. A sign of the wide acceptance of psychoanalysis and of its importance and presence in the cultural life of Argentina was given last year, when President Cristina Fernández de Kirchner and her cabinet chief took time out last April to meet for a cordial conversation in the Casa Rosada – government's Pink House – with Lacan's daughter and son-in law, when the

World Psychoanalysis Association was convening in Buenos Aires. Cartoons in local newspapers depict the caricature of an intellectual as someone who is carrying a volume of Lacan's writings under their arm. Lacan's opera magna *Ecrits* is a coffee-table book. Any cab driver can quote Freud with accuracy and elucidate opaque Lacanian dictums with enough skill to then be able to use them with precision and flair, and thus drop "the woman does not exist but if she were to exist she would be you," in their *piropos*, the flirtatious admiring catcalls addressed to women that thrive on the streets of Latin America. The psychoanalytic terminology continues to expand everyday language, and most women who are called "hysteric" take it as praise, following Lacan's idea that hysteria is not just a pathology but rather the paradigm of the speaking-being, and that which, above all, puts desire into motion. This permeability of psychoanalysis also accounts for the neologism "histeriquiar" (from hysteria), which means to flirt – no crippling pathology at stake here. Argentinean culture freely associates with the productions of Freud and Lacan.

To add one last recent example of how ingrained psychoanalysis is in Argentinean culture: in order to increase its readership, *La Nación*, one of Argentina's main newspapers, offered along with each Friday's paper a new volume of Freud's complete works at a discount. It would be hard to imagine the *New York Times* using this strategy for its promotion.

One remarkable feature is that in Argentina when one says that psychoanalysis is popular, it also means "for the people." Psychoanalysis is not just for Argentina's moneyed classes; many psychoanalysts in the state medical system offer treatment at nominal fees. And while a few private health plans may not pay for psychoanalysis, most insurance programs cover dozens of sessions a year.

In Argentina, one sees alive and well Freud's commitment to the treatment of the poor and the working classes, as documented by Elizabeth Danto's 2007 book *Freud's Free Clinics: Psychoanalysis and Social Justice 1918 1938*. While some of the top analysts here charge hundreds of dollars per session, in Argentina many work on a sliding scale in accordance with their patients' incomes, offering sessions for as little as $15 an hour. Public hospitals offer psychoanalytic treatment at very low costs or free. In Argentina, even the poor can afford an unconscious.

Respect for psychoanalysis extends to other realms as well. It is embedded in various state institutions; parents of children at public schools upon being asked to attend meetings regarding their child's behavior, for instance, are sometimes surprised to learn that one of first discussions is with a psychoanalyst employed by the school system. How can we account for this?

The strong Freudian tradition that dates back to the beginning of the 20th century cannot fully account for the widespread diffusion, acceptance and popularization of psychoanalysis. Even when in Argentina Freudian thinking grew independently, avoiding the narrowing of the medical model, this healthy development cannot account for the monumental presence of psychoanalysis in the culture. This development is very different from what took place in the United States, where psychoanalysis became a very lucrative (Hale, 1995) medical sub-specialty (Sherry Turkle, 1992), completely divorced from politics and seemingly impermeable to the pressures of history. One could argue that it was the medicalization of American psychoanalysis that brought along a cleansing of ideology and political content. Its seeming neutrality is obviously political and ideologically loaded, but reveals not just ideological naivety but also something that runs against the grain of the Freudian experience. The politicizing of psychoanalysis in the US has been amply documented by historians such as Nathan Hale (1995) and Russell Jacoby (1986.) Freud could not have been more opposed to this development and his between-wars political activism found resonances in the land of tango.

Mariano Plotkin, author of *Freud in the Pampas: The Emergence and Development of a Psychoanalytic Culture in Argentina*, knows his subject first-hand. Back in the 1960s, his parents sent him to an analyst four times a week when he was only 6 years old. Mr. Plotkin suggests one reason that psychoanalysis began flourishing here in the 1950s and 1960s was Argentines' longing for a private haven away from an increasingly conflict-ridden political sphere. Even tough military officers in Argentina sometimes sound like grief counsellors. Mr. Plotkin recalls that in 1995, when the army chief of staff apologized for the military's responsibility for countless murders and human rights abuses committed from 1976 to 1983, he spoke of "working through" the mourning process and coping with "unconscious traumas." For Plotkin, psychoanalysis replaced politics and was reduced to culture. We saw that the program taught in the University for the Career of psychology was heavily influenced by psychoanalysis; in the 1960s and 1970s psychoanalysis was incorporated in the theoretical artillery of the left. Even the military dictatorship established in 1976 did not prevent the evolution of psychoanalysis. The junta closed the National Congress, imposed censorship, banned trade unions and brought state and municipal government under military control. A brutal campaign against suspected dissidents was initiated and hundreds of clandestine detention camps set up, where thousands of people were jailed and tortured. The censorship concerned the banning of the teaching of history, reducing geography and forbidding modern mathematics because set theory is non-axiomatic. But one potentially revolutionary modality of thinking survived undetected.

One peculiar phenomenon specific to Argentina is the popularity of Jacques Lacan, the so-called Gongora of psychoanalysis, whose obscure style calls up that of the Spanish Baroque lyric poet. The strong presence of Lacanian thought in Argentina cannot be accounted for by the local healthy Freudianism. Nor can it be explained by the predominance of France as a cultural model. Lacan may be known as the French Freud, but there are more Lacanians in Buenos Aires than in Paris.

Lacanian thought started to develop in Argentina in the 1960s, in the context of a strong psychoanalytic movement, described by Elisabeth Roudinesco as very pluralist, never aligned with one doctrine in particular. Its eclectic spirit allowed for its inscription in a wide social and political frame, be it Marxist, socialist or reformist. Whereas Lacan had already been mentioned in 1936 in an article by an

Argentine psychiatrist, Emilio Pizarro Crespo, it was only 30 years later that Lacan was truly introduced, to be more precise in 1964, thanks to Oscar Massotta, a young self-taught Sartrean philosopher, an intellectual beacon for many.

Argentina was not indifferent to the French events of the spring of 1968 and the reverberations of students' revolts affected the very structure of the IPA institutions and radically transformed the training, opening psychoanalysis to social issues. By the 1970s, Latin America was already the most powerful Freudian continent in the world, its numbers rivaling the United States' American Psychoanalytic Association (APSaA). Perhaps as a response, around this time the International Psychoanalytic Association divided the world in a very bizarre manner:

1. North of the Mexican frontier.
2. South of the Mexican frontier.
3. The rest of the world.

Jacques Derrida would denounce this geopolitical division in a text of 1981 and talk about a fourth zone, the Latin America of psychoanalysis in which psychoanalysis could coexist with torture and other human rights violations. At the IPA congress in New York in 1979, the group condemned the repressive practices, disappearances, tortures and murders being committed under the military dictatorship in Argentina, with a listing of professional colleagues and family members who were among the "disappeared." Its president, Edward Joseph, however, called the atrocities that were denounced "rumors."

In 1973, Peron returned from exile to Argentina and to power, and named his new wife, Isabelita, vice-president. She would later sign the creation of the triple A (Argentine Anticommunist Alliance), a regime of state terror and persecution. In 1976, a military coup replaced Isabelita, who had become president after the death of her husband, and the country was led by a junta presided by Jorge Rafael Videla, which installed one of the most brutal regimes in Latin America: 30,000 people were assassinated and tortured; they are called *desaparecidos*. In the name of the "Christian West" the armed forces decided to eliminate the Freudianism and Marxism that "corrupted" and "degenerated" society – one general called Marx and Freud "intellectual criminals." Persecution was anonymous and silent, filtering to the very heart of subjectivity.

Some psychoanalysts collaborated with the dictatorship, others were murdered; some were able to leave the country, while the rest lay low, continuing to work in their private practice, living in fear, shame and guilt. Between 1976 and 1983, psychoanalysts and psychologists who were on the left, who were Marxist, or who participated in progressive types of treatment such as group therapies or therapeutic communities, which in the eyes of the dictatorship were seen as "subversive" or "communist," were forced to go into exile or were tortured and killed. For instance, in 1978, Beatriz Perosio, President of the Buenos Aires Association of Psychologists, was kidnapped, tortured and killed. The biggest number of university students "disappeared" was in the department of psychology.

How did Lacanian thought manage to progress in this repressive, bloody context? Lacanism is a subversive counter-culture. Was it allowed because of the seemingly esoteric considerations about mathemes, sexuation formulas, the signifier and other opaque jargon? Why was it dismissed or forgotten by the regime? The terrorism of state was very shrewd – forbidding the teaching of geography and history because they are obviously political but also the teaching of modern mathematics including set theory because non axiomatic math teaches you to think and not accept ready-made statements.

Let us not forget that Lacan, was rather an active counter-culture figure, a so-called intellectual hero who played an active role in the events on May 1968 in France but kept a healthy dose of skepticism facing the student revolts. Lacan got involved actively in politics but there is something in Lacan that cannot be reduced to politics. Lacanism in Argentina flourished under a bloody dictatorship, during the so-called "dirty war" years. People studied the work of Lacan in growing networks of small study groups, away from the university. In 1980, Lacan went to Venezuela where he met hundreds of Spanish speaking followers, whom he named "LacanoAmericans." With the return of democracy in 1983, psychoanalysis, and Lacanism in particular, expanded even more. Lacan became the reference to everyone who wanted to get involved in clinical practice. It was at that time that Lacan began to be taught in the psychology departments of all universities. Currently, there are over 100 Lacanian psychoanalytic groups and associations in Argentina.

Lacan's provocative thesis that "The unconscious is structured like a language" means that the psychoanalytic subject is immersed in a universe ruled by desire and determined by a social order ushered in by language acquisition. If the formation of symptoms results from the singular structure of the subject's individual and cultural history, Lacanian psychoanalysis will be concerned with what meaning is betrayed by signs stemming from the social structure. In other words, by making symptoms readable, psychoanalysis deciphers the message of symptoms both at a subjective and societal level. It brokers an integration of the social and psychological realms.

I will argue that Lacanian psychoanalysis flourished in Argentina because it integrates the social; it makes the unconscious political. This is what makes psychoanalysis so popular and pertinent in Latin America.

Psychoanalysis is not just fully politics nor can it be reduced to culture. A case in point is the recent controversy around the Freud exhibit at the Library of Congress which seems to show that in the US Freud's contribution has been reduced to culture, as the title of the exhibit illustrates – "Sigmund Freud: Conflict and Culture." The exhibit effectively reduced Freud to a cultural phenomenon; he became a star or an idol, comparable to Andy Warhol or John F. Kennedy. However, conflict crept back into the items exhibited, subtly and silently, at least through quotes of followers and detractors. Their comments, spread over the walls, appeared to have been chosen for their timidity rather than for brash condemnations or lavish praise. Thus, in this context it was a surprise to discover

Lacan's famous last phrase, from the 1980 Caracas conference, a little more than a year before his death: "*C'est à vous d'être lacanien, moi je suis freudien*" ("It is up to you to be Lacanian, as for myself I am a Freudian"). Among the exhibit's misfires and parapraxes one reads after Lacan's quote, ominously: "no date." In the eternal present of a symptomatic suspension, Lacan's presence is acknowledged but left outside history. As with Argentinian history, that famous quote has been put into question by no less than the organizer of that conference, Diana Rabinovich, who swears she never heard Lacan say that and could not find it in the recordings.

We can historize Lacan's role both in France and Argentina. What was called in France the Marxist Spring, in Argentina was the Freudian Spring. In Argentina, Lacan had a peculiar impact that can also explain its emergence in other Latin American countries. One of the most complex post-colonial heritages in Latin America is a twisted relation to the law. One could even talk of a void in the law. Without becoming a religious discourse (which is what happened with those who followed the APA and IPA model, as was the case in the US), Lacanian psychoanalysis offers a space where the subject is confronted with the law, not the state law, but rather the law of desire. State violence and corruption in Latin America expose the precariousness of state law. In every psychoanalytic cure, each analysand has to renounce the tyranny of *jouissance* and choose the law of desire.

There is violence in psychoanalysis. It is the violence of paying with *jouissance*, of yielding a morsel of enjoyment and renouncing to the mixture of pain and pleasure granted by symptoms. The law of desire requires such sacrifice, and in this manner differs from state law. In a country like Argentina in which corruption is rampant, the mafia, unlike in Italy or Japan, has not created a counter-power. Even the mafia is not organized enough to offer a counterbalance. Psychoanalysis in Argentina appears to be treating the effects of its violent history, a history which now has morphed in democratic times from government terror to a widespread situation of what has been called "insecurity," meaning the population lives terrorized by a constant fear of crimes and misdemeanors. Psychoanalysis may appear to be treating a symptom, but it may well be maintaining a sense of coherence or even sanity – more unconscious, less terror.

References

Danto, E. (2007). *Freud's Free Clinics: Psychoanalysis and Social Justice 1918–1938*. New York: Columbia University Press.

Hale, N. (1995). *The Rise and Crisis of Psychoanalysis in the United States: Freud and the Americans, 1917–1985*. New York: Oxford University Press.

Jacoby, R. (1983). *The Repression of Psychoanalysis: Otto Fenichel and the Political Freudians*. Chicago: University of Chicago Press.

Plotkin, M. (2002). *Freud in the Pampas: The Emergence and Development of a Psychoanalytic Culture in Argentina*. Stanford, CA: Stanford University Press.

Turkle, S. (1992). *Psychoanalytic Politics: Jacques Lacan and the French Revolution* (2nd edn.). New York: Free Association Books.

INDEX

For Product Safety Concerns and Information please contact our EU representative GPSR@taylorandfrancis.com Taylor & Francis Verlag GmbH, Kaufingerstraße 24, 80331 München, Germany